Neurology

FROM THE CLASSROOM TO THE EXAM ROOM

Jeffrey W. Clark, D.O.

Associate Professor
Department of Medicine
Texas A&M College of Medicine
College Station, Texas
Senior Staff & Vice Chairman
Department of Neurology
Scott & White Hospital/Clinic
Temple, Texas

SELECTED ARTWORK BY:

Jim Abel
Marion, Iowa

Wolters Kluwer | Lippincott Williams & Wilkins
Health
Philadelphia • Baltimore • New York • London
Buenos Aires • Hong Kong • Sydney • Tokyo

Acquisitions Editor: Frances DeStefano
Managing Editor: Leanne McMillan
Project Manager: Fran Gunning
Manufacturing Manager: Ben Rivera
Design Coordinator: Risa Clow
Compositor: Aptara, Inc.
Printer: RR Donnelley–Crawfordsville

Library of Congress Cataloging-in-Publication Data

Clark, Jeffrey W.
  Clinical neurology : from the classroom to the exam room / Jeffrey W. Clark.
    p. ; cm.
  Includes bibliographical references and index.
  ISBN-13: 978-0-7817-7395-9
  ISBN-10: 0-7817-7395-4
 1. Neurologic examination. I. Title.
  [DNLM: 1. Nervous System Diseases—diagnosis. 2. Case Reports. 3. Neurologic
Examination—methods. 4. Physician-Patient Relations. WL 141 C593c 2007]
  RC348.C53 2007
  616.8′0475—dc22

                                                              2007013860

        Care has been taken to confirm the accuracy of the information presented and to describe generally accepted practices. However, the authors, editors, and publisher are not responsible for errors or omissions or for any consequences from application of the information in this book and make no warranty, expressed or implied, with respect to the currency, completeness, or accuracy of the contents of the publication. Application of this information in a particular situation remains the professional responsibility of the practitioner.
        The authors, editors, and publisher have exerted every effort to ensure that drug selection and dosage set forth in this text are in accordance with current recommendations and practice at the time of publication. However, in view of ongoing research, changes in government regulations, and the constant flow of information relating to drug therapy and drug reactions, the reader is urged to check the package insert for each drug for any change in indications and dosage and for added warnings and precautions. This is particularly important when the recommended agent is a new or infrequently employed drug.
        Some drugs and medical devices presented in this publication have Food and Drug Administration (FDA) clearance for limited use in restricted research settings. It is the responsibility of the health care provider to ascertain the FDA status of each drug or device planned for use in their clinical practice.
        To purchase additional copies of this book, call our customer service department at (800) 638-3030 or fax orders to (301) 223-2320. International customers should call (301)223-2300.
        Visit Lippincott Williams & Wilkins on the Internet: at LWW.com. Lippincott Williams & Wilkins customer service representatives are available from 8:30 am to 6 pm, EST.

                                            10 9 8 7 6 5 4 3 2 1

Contents

Dedication

This book is dedicated to the memory of Dr. Alan Follender, our good friend and former department chairman. His career and life ended prematurely several years ago after a devastating head injury. An avid golfer, his unique persona was partially captured in this caricature, respectfully presented to him by one of his former students. He framed and proudly displayed the sketch in the neurology department for years. Dr. Follender's love and enthusiasm for teaching medical students and residents lives on and continues to grow in the department he built at Scott & White Hospital/Clinic in Temple, Texas, during more than 25 years of service.

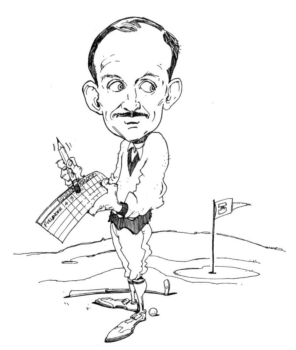

Alan Follender, MD

Abbreviations

ACA: anterior cerebral artery
ALS: amyotrophic lateral sclerosis
CNS: central nervous system
CT: computed tomography
CK: creatine kinase
DTR: deep tendon reflex
EEG: electroencephalogram (electroencephalography)
EMG: electromyography
MCA: middle cerebral artery
MRI: magnetic resonance imaging
NMJ: neuromuscular junction
TIA: transient ischemic attack
TSH: thyroid-stimulating hormone

Introduction

"I guess it's not lumbar radiculopathy."

This particular clinical impression was offered by an enthusiastic fourth-year medical student and refers to a patient who actually did, in fact, suffer from lumbar radiculopathy. Indeed, this diagnosis was confirmed by clinical history, physical exam, neuroimaging, and electromyography. However, the patient initially reported severe pain that seemed to be shooting *up* his leg, *not down*, which led the medical student to doubt the diagnosis. This bright young student's prior experience with lumbar radiculopathy was limited to a single written case study that described pain radiating *down* the limb.

As we are reminded frequently, most patients do not read the textbooks (i.e., "follow the rules"), and each person presents with a unique story. This represents a challenge for those learning clinical neurology. There is an immense body of detailed information that is

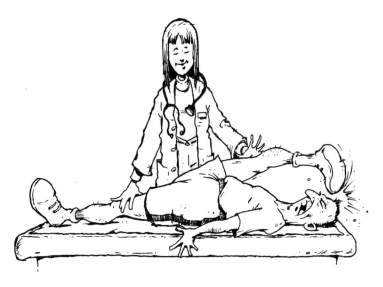

"Do you notice any discomfort when I do this?"

absorbed by first- and second-year medical students (including neuroanatomy and neurophysiology) that must eventually be organized and applied to each individual patient. This transition to clinical neurology can, at times, seem overwhelming because subjective descriptions are the norm, and the nervous system accounts for so much function. Students and residents are acutely aware that being able to recognize muscle fiber ultrastructure under a microscope or memorize a list of types of myopathy does little for those who are not yet able to diagnose myopathy presumptively based on their clinical history and examination.

This text is designed to help students and physicians bridge the wide chasm that exists between the classroom and the exam room. It offers useful principles and a reliable "system" to help navigate through this challenging and exciting transition. Once learned, the system is simple enough that it should become more or less automatic. The information will also serve as a guide to clinicians who want to teach students and residents an organized approach to clinical neurology.

Many of the paragraphs begin with quotes such as "*It must be a stroke.*" This quote, in particular, reflects one of the more common incorrect diagnoses offered by residents and medical students early on in their neurology training. Stroke is often incorrectly blamed for vague or difficult to explain symptoms—ranging from confusion to malaise—if another etiology is not evident at first glance. You may have already found that this is the case, and will soon learn how to avoid this and other common pitfalls. Many of the paragraphs from each chapter are preceded by similar quotes taken from actual physicians in training, patients, and staff. They are followed by a brief commentary to stress important principles. This format was not chosen to be sarcastic, but to interest you and hopefully strike a chord of familiarity with something you may have heard, thought, or even said before.

Again, this system is meant to serve as an essential foundation. For a more detailed review of neuroanatomy and specific clinical conditions, or for a discussion of the complete neurologic exam, please liberally consult the suggested readings that are listed at the end of the text. Have fun testing the system, and learn as you go.

Your Approach to the Neurologic Patient

WHERE DO YOU START?

You need to have an approach to patients with potential neurologic problems that is both efficient and accurate. A reliable method of evaluating each problem will consistently provide needed direction and prevent unnecessary diversions. Read on to find out the best place to begin and how to proceed when faced with a neurologic problem.

"If it moves when it shouldn't—it's a seizure, but if it doesn't move when it should— then it's a stroke."

Using limited resources and skill, one can occasionally make a correct diagnosis by applying an oversimplified rule or two. When a medical student or resident was "lucky" enough to stumble across a correct diagnosis using such a rule, our former chairman, the sage Dr. Alan Follender, would wryly declare that "Even a blind three-legged dog occasionally finds a bone." This "shoot from the hip" approach is certainly fast, but it will not be reliable on a day-to-day basis. This is especially the case when evaluating potential neurologic problems.

The basic four-step approach is preferred and essential to clinical neurology. Experienced neurologists go through the same steps

1

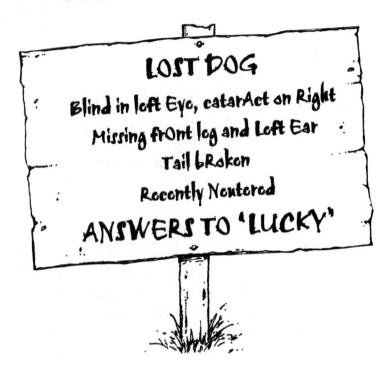

so seamlessly that the physician-in-training only sees the end product, a correct diagnosis. Using this systematic method initially requires some patience and practice. However, it reliably provides much-needed direction from the start, and helps save time, effort, and expense in the long run:

1. *Where* in the NeurAxis is the problem/dysfunction? **(location)**
2. *What* could the problem be at this level in this patient? **(differential)**
3. Which *test* would be useful to confirm this initial impression? **(confirmation)**
4. Is *therapy* indicated or available at this point for this problem? **(treatment)**

Answering these questions in sequence allows for a *logical* and efficient progression from the patient's reported symptom(s) to the appropriate test or intervention/treatment. The organized clinician will waste much less time, order fewer superfluous tests, and avoid unnecessary digressions. The majority of the information discussed in this book will direct the clinician in efficiently answering the first and most important (essential) question: **Where** *is the problem?*

"I have this guy in the ER who is weak. Should I get the brain CT with or without contrast?"

It has been said that our most expensive tool as physicians is the pen. Laboratory and/or radiologic testing should be based on a solid clinical impression derived from the interview and examination, not on a single reported symptom. This is especially important in neurology because a number of distinct areas (levels) may be tested by a variety of different technologies. Reflexively ordering a cranial CT scan on all patients with ill-defined subjective "weakness" will eventually lead to confusion (on the physician's part), delayed care, and increased costs. Be sure not to skip **step one!**

"Should we start heparin on every patient with stroke?"

Years ago, one of our residents confidently declared that the use of intravenous heparin in patients with ischemic infarct of the brain was "part of the protocol." This practice had, in fact, become so common that it was assumed to be part of a protocol or "cookbook" approach to managing stroke at our institution. However, we were never actually able to locate this written set of instructions, and medical research has since shown that the use of heparin in these cases is not usually indicated.

House officers as a group are often fond of written protocols. Indeed, they can provide a strong sense of certainty within an otherwise unpredictable and sometimes hectic environment. However, medical knowledge and technology have evolved so rapidly since the mid-1990s that many algorithms have quickly become obsolete. Technology and research have also allowed for a greater understanding of nervous system disease in recent years. One might assume that this has made clinical neurology easier or possibly less important. However, with more available tests and treatment options to choose from, the clinical neurologic assessment is actually becoming ***more*** critical, not less so. We are now required to diagnose and treat certain patients much sooner (e.g., using thrombolysis to treat ischemic stroke) and in a more cost-effective manner than ever before (i.e., avoiding unnecessary tests).

This book is designed to help you become more efficient at identifying **where** the nervous system dysfunction is based on a limited number of important signs and symptoms (i.e., step one). To start using this method, all you need is a basic working knowledge of the nervous system. Anyone who has taken an anatomy course is familiar with each level of the nervous system (NeurAxis), including the cerebral hemispheres, spinal cord, and peripheral nerves. Using this knowledge as a foundation, you will quickly develop a framework to help sort through the levels efficiently based on available clinical information.

Step one is simply defining the most likely *level* of nervous system dysfunction, or **where** the problem is. This is referred to as "bracketing" and is different than trying to "localize the lesion" with pinpoint accuracy. It is simply a matter of learning to recognize certain common patterns associated with each level. For instance, unilateral limb weakness in a "pyramidal pattern" would suggest a cerebral hemisphere abnormality, especially if accompanied by ipsilateral facial weakness, sensory loss, or visual field change. Conversely, bilateral ascending paresis with sensory loss and diminished muscle stretch reflexes would be suggestive of peripheral neuropathy (possibly Guillain-Barré syndrome if symptoms are rapidly progressive). Such patients must be triaged and treated urgently, but the appropriate confirmatory laboratory tests, clinical management, and prognosis are quite different. The stark contrast between these two examples in terms of diagnosis and treatment helps illustrate the necessity of starting with a correct anatomic diagnosis.

Step two in the process is determining the most likely cause (etiology) of the problem once the level of involvement has been identified. In other words, **what** is the problem at the defined level? Considerations include infarction, infection, inflammation, trauma, or metabolic (see CITTEN DVM in Chapter 5). Your "educated guess" will be based on the patient's clinical profile and history given the level of nervous system affected. This particular step requires a bit more clinical experience and knowledge, and is always dependent on first accurately identifying the level of dysfunction (step one). For example, you recall that unilateral pyramidal pattern limb weakness

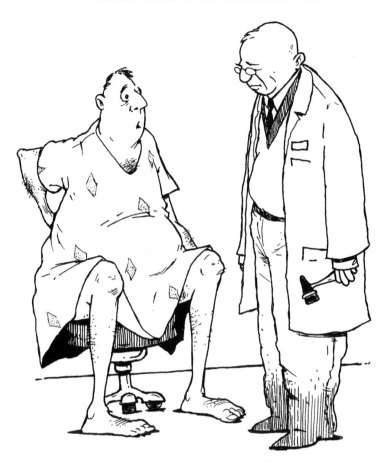

"Doc, my back is killing me. Do you think it could be some kind of brain tumor?"

with facial involvement suggests contralateral cerebral hemisphere dysfunction. If this pattern of findings suddenly occurred in a 70-year-old hypertensive man, then stroke would be highest on your differential and urgent CT imaging would be ordered. Conversely, if your patient was a 20-year-old woman and had similar findings that had progressed more slowly, then multiple sclerosis would be higher on your differential. In her case, outpatient MRI of the brain might be the best option.

Resist the urge to "shoot from the hip" by immediately making a clinical diagnosis and/or ordering a lab test without first identifying the level involved. Draw your pen from its holster only *after* determining the likely level(s) of dysfunction. You will then be able to confidently order appropriate tests based on the suspected etiology when considering the patient's unique clinical profile.

"Was that a true story?"

In the film *Good Will Hunting,* psychiatrist Sean Maguire *(Robin Williams)* counsels Will Hunting *(Matt Damon),* who possesses the intellect and memory of a genius. While sweeping floors as a janitor at the Massachusetts Institute of Technology, Will Hunting easily solves complex math equations left on the blackboard for graduate students to ponder. He even quotes various authors by page and paragraph from memory. No, it is not a true story, and most of us unfortunately do not exhibit that kind of computerlike ability to memorize and manipulate an almost unlimited number of random facts.

A computer program (or individual like this with a photographic memory) could theoretically remember all possible diseases and compare each patient's symptoms and signs with those expected for each condition. This memory-intensive "digital" approach requires near-perfect recall and extensive clinical experience, not to mention the ability to accurately perform an examination. It quickly "breaks down" when the physician is short on time, experience, or an internal hard drive. Surprisingly, this is the method used by many medical students and residents to evaluate neurologic problems. As we say in Texas, "That dog won't hunt." As practicing clinicians, we generally do not have the time (or memory) to approach clinical problems like that, and computer programs are not yet able to collect the necessary data by interview and examination.

A much simpler and effective approach to neurology is to conceptualize the nervous system as a set of **distinct areas** with functional limits instead of myriad tracts and nuclei. The nervous system can easily be separated into these levels based on location and function. We refer to this as the *NeurAxis.* Be patient, and read on. You will soon learn how to compare and contrast the patient's history and exam findings with the limits of function associated with each level. This logical method places emphasis on first identifying **where** the problem is located, and is inherently more organized and less memory intensive than the "digital" approach. It can be mastered quickly, even by those with limited clinical experience, and then used as a reliable framework on which to build. You will see that it is a much more manageable task than trying to learn and memorize hundreds of separate neurologic conditions one by one.

The NeurAxis can be separated functionally and anatomically into ten distinct but interactive levels. Because you already know these from your basic anatomy course, it will be easy for you to begin thinking about neurologic problems in terms of the level affected:

1. Cerebral hemispheres
2. Brainstem
3. Cerebellum
4. Spinal cord
5. Anterior horn cells/cranial nerve nuclei
6. Nerve root
7. Plexus
8. Peripheral nerve (named)
9. Neuromuscular junction
10. Muscle

"All of the sudden she couldn't talk."

This patient's problem illustrates how a single clinical symptom or sign can serve as your ally in identifying the NeurAxis level affected. You know that the centers for language function are located in the dominant cerebral hemisphere, which is on the left 95% of the time (occasionally on the right in left-handed patients). Someone who suddenly loses the ability to process language (communicate verbally) almost certainly has a problem in this region, with stroke being the most common cause in patients who are elderly. Regardless of the patient's age, we can bank on a left hemisphere abnormality as the cause of language problems based on known function at that level of the axis. Likewise, we know from clinical experience that each of the ten NeurAxis levels accounts for a certain amount and pattern of neurologic function. Therefore, dysfunction or damage at any of these levels results in a relatively distinct pattern of **signs** and *symptoms*. For instance, a problem in the cervical spinal cord could cause weakness of all four limbs, but not of the face. A problem in the cerebellum is associated with ataxia, but not sensory loss. As you can see, much of

Doris had to wait 2 months for her neurology appointment, so she wanted to make the most of it.

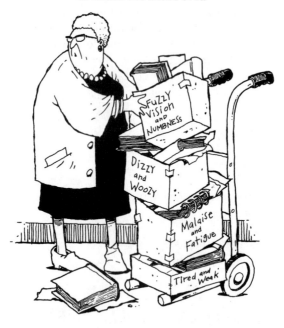

"I've kept up with most of my symptoms."

this is intuitively obvious if you can resist the urge to jump to a specific diagnosis.

Knowing which questions to ask (i.e., the **clinical history**) and what to look for (i.e., the **examination**) are the most important issues that allow us to quickly and reliably narrow the possibilities. This diagnostic approach is called **bracketing,** which means identifying the general *region* of the nervous system that is affected. It is much easier than making a "pinpoint precise" anatomic diagnosis and simpler than making a specific clinical diagnosis. You do not need to try to define the exact spinal level (e.g., T-5) or cranial nerve nucleus affected (e.g., mesencephalic nucleus of V). Once you know enough to suspect a thoracic cord problem because of bilateral lower extremity weakness with incontinence, then imaging of this area can be confidently ordered. Conversely, a different region would be imaged if you suspected a brainstem lesion based on the presence of crossed sensory or motor findings (one side of the face and opposite side of the body affected). These distinct recognizable patterns illustrate the potential straightforwardness of this approach. As you can see, it places emphasis on comprehension and not memorization. Because patients often present with a variety of symptoms, it is necessary to have a consistent starting point and sense of direction to help guide the assessment. You should already have some familiarity with each level, and this will serve as your framework. You will be able to build on this knowledge base easily with each patient you see and every paragraph you read from this point on.

The NeurAxis system is presented in chart form in Chapter 5. You may want to look ahead and take a quick glance at the chart before reading Chapters 3 and 4, which discuss important concepts and issues related to performing a useful neurologic history and examination. Carry a copy of the chart with you to the clinic or hospital and look it over when discussing neurologic problems. Soon neurology will make sense, and you will not need to refer to your notes at all!

2

The Clinical History

**GETTING THE IMPORTANT INFORMATION
YOU NEED EFFICIENTLY**

*W*hether *you are still in the classroom and fairly new
to patient care or are an experienced clinician, you
already know that some basic information must be
obtained from the patient (or historian) before the evaluation can begin. This is especially the case in neurology
because the nervous system covers so much ground (literally head to toe) and is responsible for so much function,
ranging from autonomic function to strength to cognition. This being the case, you can extract more information with greater efficiency if you remain aware of important issues and principles that are unique to neurology.*

"Well, did you ask?"

Prior to developing a natural sense of direction through clinical
experience, students and residents will often forget to ask about a
variety of important items during the history. This, I am told,
becomes a great source of stress for students and residents when
their attending physician needs the unavailable information to
make a diagnosis (which they invariably do from time to time).
However, when you use the NeurAxis as a **roadmap**, the right
questions will come naturally as you begin to bracket the patient's
problem to a particular region. The diagnostic possibilities will be

narrowed down efficiently as you use your history-taking skills to scan the NeurAxis from **head to toe**. When distal weakness is reported, you will automatically ask about associated sensory loss and paresthesias. These symptoms combined with diminished muscle stretch reflexes (which you will also remember to check) suggest a problem of the peripheral nervous system (e.g., peripheral neuropathy). Taking a *useful* history is not a matter of collecting a long list of random facts in case the attending physician asks. It is simply a matter of compiling relevant information, including the **distribution** and **type** of symptoms, so you are confidently guided to the level of the lesion. It is a skill that improves with experience, so be patient.

"I just didn't know where to start."

Visualize a skilled linebacker intensely scanning up and down the offensive line and backfield looking for clues that will help identify the next play. You likewise will be **scanning** up and down the nervous system (NeurAxis) to determine where the "action" is. Start with the chief complaint, and then pick a reasonable level and go up and then down the axis from that point with your questions.

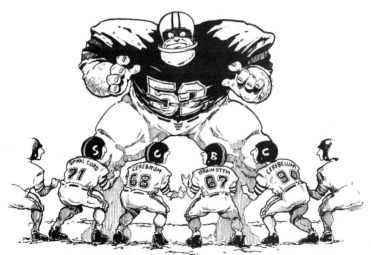

**Quickly scan up and down the NeurAxis,
from the cerebral hemispheres down to the muscle.**

If the complaint is trouble swallowing, you might start at the brainstem level, asking about diplopia, speech difficulty, and balance trouble. Then go up to the cerebral hemispheres and ask about any seizures, language dysfunction, or cognitive changes. Soon you will work your way back down through the brainstem to the spinal cord and eventually to the neuromuscular junction. The list of potential diseases is long, but the NeurAxis is finite and well defined. There are a relatively small number of "high-yield" symptoms that have proven to be more useful when sorting out the level affected, and these are discussed in detail later in this chapter. In terms of where to actually begin, a tentative hypothesis based on the chief complaint is usually a good starting point, and the NeurAxis is your roadmap. When you use the NeurAxis levels as a guide, the most important questions will come naturally, and all of the information you collect will be useful.

Before you even have a chance to perform the formal examination, your initial clinical impression will be based primarily on the **symptoms** endorsed by the patient and his or her unique **story** surrounding the illness. If you try to proceed without these essential elements, which are vital to comprising a good history, you may be swimming in a sea of uncertainty when it comes to performing your exam. You will inevitably find yourself ordering unnecessary lab studies. However, when armed with a reliable history, the clinical examination and relevant laboratory tests can be performed with the confidence that comes with a true sense of direction. Extracting a history from a textbook case is easy, but obtaining one from a patient can be quite challenging. The following paragraphs include some of the more important concepts related to performing the clinical history that will help you out immediately.

"I'm weak."

This patient's particular situation was confusing to the resident because the tests ordered for evaluation of his reported **"weakness"** were normal. These included EMG, lumbar spine MRI, serum CK, and TSH. Furthermore, the clinical examination actually revealed **normal motor power**. There was no muscle weakness at all! This type of discrepancy in reported symptoms and objective examination findings is common. Part of the reason is that patients usually report their symptoms in lay terms that make sense to them, but these do not always correlate with our medical terminology. More pointed questioning during the history should ferret this out. In this particular case, additional clinical information obtained during a more focused history revealed that the patient had noticeable trouble ambulating. This was actually caused by gait unsteadiness (ataxia), which he reported as "weakness."

Gait instability is often reported as "weakness" because patients may feel like their legs are "giving way." However, patients sometimes label true weakness (loss of motor power) as **"falling spells"** or **"dizziness"** because of difficulty with ambulation. **"Numbness"** is a term used by patients to describe a variety of problems, including tingling or burning (paresthesias), loss of sensation (true numbness), trouble controlling an arm or leg (limb ataxia), or even loss of strength (weakness).

When a clinical diagnosis remains elusive, an inefficient approach would be to continue ordering a variety of lab tests until an abnormality surfaces. A better method would be to start over from the beginning with a focused **history**. Although it may not seem efficient at that point, this usually turns out to be a time saver. As illustrated by the previous case, one of the initial challenges in taking a history is translating the patient's complaint(s) into accurate and useful medical descriptions prior to formulating a presumptive diagnosis. Patients definitely want to help us identify their problem. We just need to take the time necessary to understand what they are really saying to us. This is a valuable investment because the information directs both the examination and the laboratory testing.

"Coma!"

Coma is a potentially emergent condition that can strike fear even in the heart of well-trained house officers, sometimes leading to a flurry of tests. The etiology of coma is often hidden in (or established by) the **clinical history**. Physicians in all specialties will tell you that if you do not have a fairly good idea of what the problem is after taking the history, the next step is not to order a test but to go back and take another history. Evaluating a comatose patient often proves this rule. In situations where other sources must be contacted, a good history may seem like the most difficult portion of the evaluation to complete, but the investment in time can be invaluable.

If you discover, for instance, that this coma patient is a construction worker who fell from a three-story building, then the presumptive diagnosis of head trauma would lead to an urgent brain imaging study. If, instead, he is a known diabetic, then testing blood sugar and administering glucose as soon as possible may be life saving. Lumbar puncture is a test that you might perform if infection or subarachnoid hemorrhage were a concern. Many tests are available, but only one can be performed at a time, and a select few may be necessary to confirm your diagnosis when the history is clear. In addition to adding cost and time to patient care, superfluous tests can be very misleading. As one popular aphorism goes, "Two minutes of history is often worth 2 days of testing."

"I started scratching this year."

This patient was a healthy senior Olympian ("76 years young") who had been able to hold on to her long jumping title for several years running. However, this year she frequently found herself accidentally stepping past the take-off mark. This is referred to as "scratching" in track and field and disqualifies the jump. Further history revealed that she had also noticed occasional "dragging" of the same leg late in the day. The additional information helped us focus the exam, which included an extended walk up and down the corridor. On initial inspection, she appeared to be in excellent shape neurologically, but subtle abnormalities were identified after longer ambulation. A diagnosis of Parkinson disease was made, and with treatment, she was able to defend her title that year.

Patients, if specifically asked, will provide useful information by reporting problems with certain day-to-day tasks. Remember to inquire about difficulties with "activities of daily living," such as brushing teeth, buttoning a shirt, pouring a drink, playing cards, and physical recreation. If someone is able to ride a bicycle, throw a ball accurately, or jog 5 miles, then it's a good indication that strength and coordination are functionally normal. If they can run a business, pay the bills on time, plan a meal, or organize a family reunion, then cognitive function is probably quite good as well.

"But he has a very complicated neurologic history..."

This is a phrase that we commonly hear from residents and others who refer patients to us. This referring physician was almost in a panic on the phone, asking that her patient be seen immediately. The patient's complaint was right foot drop, but no further relevant information was obtained from the patient after the examiner realized that he had suffered from subarachnoid hemorrhage 20 years prior. The patient's neurologic history at that point was labeled "complicated," and the physician was not confident enough to continue with a more detailed history and exam. It turns out that 20 years ago, he had suffered from a traumatic subarachnoid hemorrhage. More recently, he noticed that his right foot would not dorsiflex well after standing from the sofa at the end of a Super Bowl party. This mild foot drop with sensory change on the dorsum of his foot was actually improving, and no treatment was necessary. He was diagnosed with mild peroneal neuropathy due to prolonged leg crossing. Two or three simple questions were enough to determine that his symptoms were not related to recurrent subarachnoid hemorrhage. Before you pick up the phone to call in a referral or a pen to write orders, ask a few relevant questions and see if the diagnosis becomes more apparent.

"My mom came to visit."

Multiple symptoms that are vague or difficult to diagnose should not, by default, be attributed to the nervous system. Stated another way, problems that are difficult to diagnose should not be attributed to a system that you find difficult to understand (i.e., the nervous system). This patient was referred for a third neurologic opinion because his long list of complaints were vague, nonspecific, and remained undiagnosed after an extensive evaluation at two other medical centers. His symptoms included general lack of energy, dizziness, insomnia, weight fluctuation, and intermittent abdominal discomfort. He and his fiancée were both very concerned because they were unable to identify any particular event or "stressor" that could have triggered these symptoms.

A thorough social history revealed that these symptoms began just after his mother had traveled to the United States from another country to meet his fiancée. He had been engaged for several months, and the wedding was looming. The woman accompanying him during the interview looked a little more than twice his age. I assumed that this was his mother (or possibly his grandmother). As it turns out, *she* was actually his fiancée, the woman his mother originally came to meet. His mother clearly did not approve of their plans to marry, but neither of them seemed to realize that this was a significant stressor for him. This important historical information helped confirm a nonneurologic diagnosis, and after dealing with the issues at hand, his symptoms quickly resolved.

"I just can't work anymore."

One of the basics of history taking 101 is to inquire about what makes a problem **worse**, what tends to make it **better**, and to ask if anything was associated in time with the **onset**. This woman was no longer able to perform her job because of hand and arm pain with associated hand tingling by the end of each workday. When asked, she described her job, which was to stretch vinyl cloth manually and attach it to boat seats with a hand stapler for 6 to 8 hours each workday. Nerve conduction tests confirmed the clinical suspicion of carpal tunnel syndrome (median neuropathy at the wrist), and with appropriate treatment, her symptoms resolved. Remember to ask about potential **exacerbating factors** such as environmental triggers, body position, physical trauma, medication changes, or other inciting events. Identifying a pattern of symptom improvement or worsening is often very helpful in diagnosing the etiology of a particular problem.

"I couldn't see anything."

Reported **loss of vision** almost always requires some clarification. Sudden complete bilateral loss of vision is rare, whereas blurring (change in acuity) is common. Patients, however, often report "loss of vision" or describe being "unable to see" when referring to a slight change in visual acuity. Other possibilities include diplopia, transient monocular blindness (amaurosis fugax), or flashing lights/colors (photopsia). A careful history and exam should be undertaken to determine which of these (if any) is the case.

Ask the patient whether **covering either eye** makes a difference; this will help determine if the change in vision is monocular (affecting one eye) or homonymous (affecting either the right or the left field of vision). **Double vision** (diplopia) can be monocular or binocular, and may be vertical or horizontal. Patients with **blurred vision**, or decreased acuity, should report trouble with reading or focusing on fine details. Any of these problems may be reported initially as "loss of vision." Sorting out the problem efficiently is important because the pathology responsible for altered vision may range in location from the cornea to the optic nerve to the occipital lobe

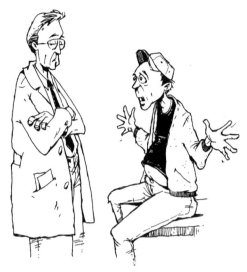

*"All of a sudden I couldn't see anything,
so I drove over here as fast as I could!"*

(and even to the brainstem in the case of binocular diplopia). The history is what helps you determine which test to order and/or which specialist to consult.

"Binocular?"

Remember that **binocular** diplopia resolves with covering either eye, while **monocular** diplopia resolves only when the affected eye is occluded. Binocular diplopia is generally due to a disturbance of ocular motility, whereas monocular diplopia suggests a problem with the eye itself. New onset dysconjugate gaze leads to binocular diplopia because the eyes are not foveating on the same object. This can be caused by a problem with one of four levels of the NeurAxis: (i) posterior fossa (brainstem or cerebellar tracts); (ii) ocular motor nerve(s) (CN 3, 4, or 6); (iii) the neuromuscular junction; or (iv) extraocular muscle(s).

Monocular diplopia implies a problem with the eye/globe somewhere from the cornea to the retina, and usually affects only one eye at a time. Sudden onset of diplopia that is monocular but bilateral is therefore suspicious for a psychiatric condition (e.g., conversion disorder or malingering). As you can see, which test is appropriate and whether one decides to call a neurologist, ophthalmologist, or psychiatrist for help rests on **anatomic diagnosis**, which is heavily dependent on the patient's description of the problem.

"I just want to be able to go back to work. I love my job."

This patient complained of severe migrating somatic pain that would affect one limb at a time, moving to another without warning from hour to hour or day to day. A number of tests had been performed prior to his neurology visit, and all were fortunately interpreted as normal. Tests included MRI of the brain and lumbar spine and nerve conduction studies. His neurologic examination was entirely normal, including strength, muscle stretch reflexes, and sensation. He had been off work for about 3 months and was about to apply for long-term disability because his sick days and vacation had been used up. He declared half a dozen times that he "just wanted to be able to go back to work" as a prison guard. It became fairly clear after allowing him to talk about his duties that his problem was job-related stress and not neurologic in origin. Clues such as this present themselves to the patient historian, so listen closely.

"I've never had headaches before."

Patients with headache and chronic somatic pain frequently experience an evolution of their pain over years to decades, and often experience different types of pain over time. Often, a change in pain will be reported as an entirely new problem, and they may even omit from their history any past significant headache or somatic pain problems. Keep this in mind as you are extracting the history. Be patient and rephrase your questions to determine if anything similar has been experienced in the past. You may need to ask about other types of headache or somatic pain several times to get the full story. Spending a bit of extra time on the history may prevent unnecessary testing, as well as the confusion and uncertainty that can follow. For instance, one study using MRI revealed an intervertebral disc abnormality in 64% of individuals without back pain, and another revealed a herniated disc in 36% of asymptomatic people ≥60 years of age. normalities on cranial MRI have been reported in a significant

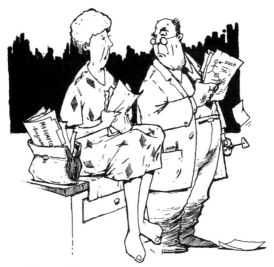

"Don't think you are going to figure out my problem that easily. I still have two more pages of symptoms to confuse you with."

number of asymptomatic volunteers. Misleading test results can often be avoided by taking a comprehensive history, sometimes for a second or even a third time.

"What's the take-home message?"

Students of medicine have a lot to learn within a relatively limited amount of time. Boiling each lesson down to a digestible "take-home message" can be very helpful. So, remember this: Don't underestimate the power of reliable clinical information. Start with a careful history, and if the diagnosis remains uncertain after your exam or lab testing, then take *another* history.

3

The Neurologic Examination

TIPS AND TECHNIQUES TO HELP IMPROVE YOUR YIELD

The neurologic exam can be fairly simple to perform and interpret if you approach it systematically as you do the history. Keep the NeurAxis in mind as you assess the patient, learn the correct method for performing each portion of the exam, and apply appropriate terminology to help avoid confusion.

"The neurologic exam was stone-cold normal."

This is what the neurologist often hears near just before detecting several subtle but significant abnormalities on his or her neurologic exam. A brief screening exam can be useful for triaging patients but may not always reveal subtle abnormalities. These incomplete exams are sometimes reported as "stone-cold normal." Remember that neurologic patients often exhibit **subtle abnormalities** that are exposed only when you focus on a particular region or "push the edge of the envelope" with regard to testing nervous system function. One of the most sensitive, albeit impractical, methods of assessing the nervous system would be to observe patients in their own environment. Watching them ride a bike, prepare a meal, balance a checkbook, or plan a vacation would all be very telling. Because this is rarely possible, simple suggestions are offered throughout this chapter to help you improve your yield in identifying and recording abnormalities on the mental status, cranial nerve, motor, and sensory portions of your exam.

"Neurologic exam was grossly normal."

The author of this particular statement knows what he found on the examination. Unfortunately, nobody else can really be certain. Almost as important as the examination is the record of it. Accurate documentation allows others to know what was done and what was found. Many who record a "grossly normal exam" will admit that they didn't actually test strength or sensation, but the patient "seemed normal" when observed during a brief encounter (sometimes from the doorway).

If muscle strength is entirely normal, then briefly list the muscles tested and record muscle power in these as normal. If your exam is incomplete, avoid the urge to label strength "pretty good throughout" or "grossly normal." Briefly note which tests were performed (e.g., gait, station, strength) and complete the exam later when time allows. Using more specific, less ambiguous terms is also helpful, so avoid generalizations and eponyms when possible. Results written

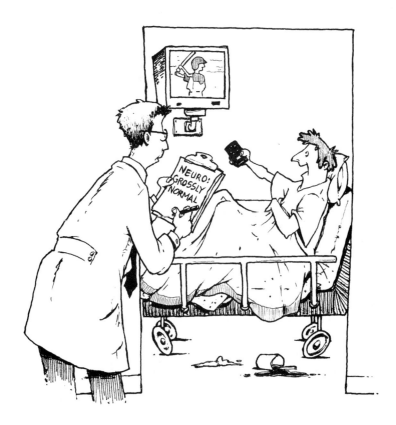

descriptively are useful for the examiner and can even be reinterpreted later by others, if necessary.

Member: secret service

Some residents refer to dermatologists, neurologists, and ophthalmologists as members of the "secret service" because few seem to inherently understand their jargon. Unfortunately, semantic confusion in medicine can be a real problem, occasionally leading to time-consuming delays in management. A good way to avoid this is to use **descriptive language** in lieu of confusing terms and misunderstood eponyms. As one of our residents added, "If eponyms impress the friends you hang out with, then maybe you should get out more." Reporting what you found in a more straightforward manner helps streamline care and avoid unnecessary delays in management.

"He had a left-sided stroke."

If you have ever written something similar, it was obvious to you at the time what you meant. However, "**left-sided stroke**" may refer to left-sided weakness (due to a right hemisphere stroke) or right-sided weakness (due to a left hemisphere stroke). In my experience, the student or resident usually means left-sided somatic weakness. If you have ever been called to reevaluate a stroke patient quickly (especially late at night when the admitting team is not present), you know the value of a precise and descriptive diagnosis. Try this next time: "Mr. Jones suffered from a right cerebral hemisphere infarct and exhibits left-sided face, arm, and leg weakness." You might even shorten it to the following when you are summarizing the patient's condition: "Right hemisphere infarct with left body weakness."

"She was stuporous yesterday but obtunded this morning."

Is it clear to you whether this patient's condition has improved or worsened over the past 24 hours? Terms like these rarely provide useful information beyond the obvious implication that the patient is not entirely normal. A simple description of the patient's condition would be much more helpful in day-to-day care and for those who may follow the examiner. The best description usually originates with a mental picture of how the patient appears to you at the time. For example, see if this description helps you more than either of the previous terms: "Ms. Doe is currently supine, intubated, and breathing spontaneously above the ventilator setting of 12 breaths per minute. She opens her eyes to vigorous shaking but not to verbal stimulation/command." Make a habit of using specific terms that add clarity, not those that tend to confuse others and obscure the clinical picture.

"Mental status seemed normal."

The mental status exam consists of more than asking a person if they can recall their name, current date, and three objects. There are more questions that need to be asked and different ways to perform the exam, depending on how the information is to be used. The **mental status exam** and "**Mini Mental State**" **exam** are not synonymous. The Mini Mental State exam is a simple standardized cognitive screening test that can be used as a research tool and in the clinic. However, it is not a particularly sensitive test of cognitive function. Many intelligent and highly educated patients may perform very well on this brief exam, even when suffering from early dementia. There are other similar brief tests of cognitive function with good inter-rater reliability that have also been copyrighted (e.g., the Short Test of Mental Status). Remember, family members may notice problems at home or in the work environment long before these types of tests are significantly abnormal, especially in highly educated patients.

For a more comprehensive picture of higher-level cognitive function, take the time to carefully interview the patient's family and/or friends. Then discuss current events, hobbies, and other interests with the patient him- or herself. Open-ended questions such as "Who runs the country?" or "What do you like to do?" allow for individuality of answers. Narrow or overgeneralized responses are common in early dementia. Asking "What's going on in the world right now?" will lead to responses such as "chaos," "wars everywhere," or "lots of trouble." With follow-up questioning, these patients are often unable to provide a description, explanation, or any significant/accurate details. "The president" may be all this patient offers when asked "Who runs the country?" Be careful not to give credit for a correct answer just because you agree with their opinion they jokingly respond, "Oh, that rascal, you know who it is…." Those functioning at a normal level will usually provide a proper name and may even spontaneously provide details related to the inner workings of a representative republic. If your patient is a sports fan, then discuss his or her favorite team. If your

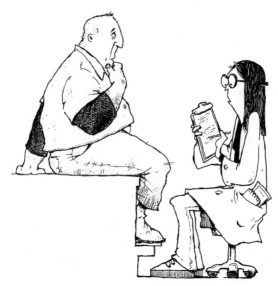

*"If you don't answer these last two questions
correctly, then I will need to count
your cortical neurons."*

patient is a gardener, then talk with him or her about plants. Patients with dementia will provide fewer details and shorter lists (e.g., types of flowers or vegetables one might grow, different animals found on a farm, or teams in a league). These and similar questions will provide much more information than the standard dementia profile and are less awkward than asking "Do you know where you are?" or "Can you tell me your full name?"

Clock drawing test

If you are interested in a screening test and not a full mental status evaluation, a very good test that assesses executive function quickly is the **clock drawing test.** It takes only a minute or two to perform, is easy to interpret, and crosses cultural and educational boundaries. Just ask the patient to draw the face of a clock with the numbers on it. Then ask them to show a specific time on the clock, such as "twenty 'til eleven" or "ten fifteen." Each number should be correctly located and evenly spaced. There should be two hands of different lengths that point at or near the correct numbers for the time indicated.

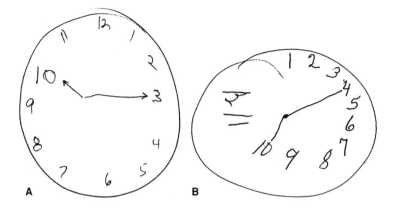

These two patients (see clocks) were asked to indicate "ten fifteen" on their clocks. You can see that patients do not need to speak English or have a formal education to draw a simple clock face. Can you easily tell which of these two is abnormal?

"I didn't have a vision card to test acuity."

Two important tests often omitted from the cranial nerve exam are visual acuity and visual fields. Patients are quick to detect and report complete loss of vision or change in acuity but may not even be aware of diminished **peripheral vision**. Loss of peripheral vision in either or both eyes can occur insidiously if progression is slow. You should check the respective **visual fields** in each eye by confrontation testing. **Visual acuity** can be reliably estimated even if you don't have a formal vision card available. Use a newspaper, magazine, or even your ID tag. Standard newsprint at half an arm's length requires about 20/40 acuity. Using a magazine or newspaper, start with the headlines or larger print and move to smaller letters or numbers based on the patient's ability. This information will be useful immediately and will help later, especially if vision changes are reported.

Pupils should be tested with the overhead lights off to allow for full dilation, and for accurate comparison of size and shape between sides. A very useful tool for examining small or minimally reactive pupils is a lighted magnifying glass. These can be purchased for a few dollars at your local drugstore. If you like to use the abbreviation "PERRLA" be sure to actually test for accommodation. You may want to simply describe size, shape, and reactivity instead. Most students realize quickly that the funduscopic exam is simple but not always easy. Seize the opportunity to practice your funduscopic exam on younger patients while the light is dimmed. This will help you develop the skill necessary to see the fundus in older patients with small pupils or mild cataract.

"I didn't watch them walk."

Deciding which portions of the exam to perform can be difficult when time is short or the patient's cooperation is limited. Two of the most useful neurologic tests overall are assessment of **walking** and **talking**. If time or other constraints prevent a complete exam, then these two will usually be at the top of your short list. Ironically, both are sometimes omitted in the hospitalized patient. In an effort to avoid "bothering" the person who appears ill or tired, a full mental

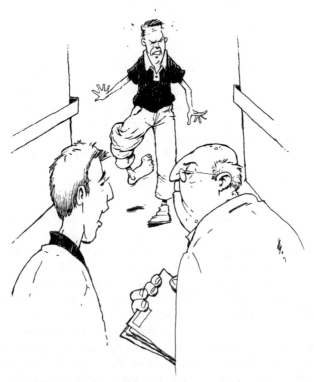

"You think he might have some kind of leg problem?"

status exam and even conversation are bypassed. Likewise, gait analysis can be cumbersome and is, therefore, often omitted when several "lines" are in place (e.g., IV, oxygen, urinary catheter).

There are several reasons that assessment of gait and station, speech, and language are so valuable. If gait appears entirely normal, then balance, lower extremity strength, and coordination are all probably good. Even minor abnormalities can affect the speed of walking, rhythm, or symmetry of movements. A substantial amount of neurologic function is also reflected in a brief verbal exchange. If the examiner is attentive, then speech, language, mentation, and even emotion can all be at least partially assessed. Learn to focus all of your attention on the patient during the interview because other problems such as subtle facial asymmetry, fluctuations in voice, fasciculations, and abnormal limb movements may be transient.

The 30-second neurologic exam

This exercise will help you hone your neurologic skills and streamline your evaluation at the same time. It will also prove to you how much information assessment of walking and talking provides. Before you formally evaluate a clinic patient with any neurologic symptom, formulate a presumptive diagnosis with limited information as follows: Note the chief complaint, and then simply watch the patient walk down the hall into the examination room. Carefully observe the patient's gate, the way he or she moves, and how he or she interacts with others along the way. At that point, you should have enough information to come up with a relatively short list of potential diagnoses. This brief encounter will provide valuable clues by helping you answer the following questions: Was the patient's gait smooth and steady with good rhythm and arm swing? Was limping, staggering, or pain evident? Were upper and lower extremity movements symmetric and coordinated? Did the patient sway, stagger, touch the wall for balance, or stop for rest? Was assistance or a walking aid necessary? How did the patient respond to the desk personnel, and was the patient attentive and conversing intelligibly with his or her family? Was the patient's speech slurred or voice hypophonic? Did the patient appear confused, tired, anxious, or happy? The information you now have will take you a long way toward a likely diagnosis.

For instance, right upper extremity adduction with elbow/wrist flexion and circumduction of the right lower extremity would suggest pyramidal predilection (upper motoneuron) weakness. If combined with ipsilateral facial weakness or paraphasic language errors, then a left cerebral hemisphere problem could be presumed (possibly cerebral infarction in the elderly patient). If, instead, the patient was limping and/or grimacing with each step, then a more peripheral problem may be suspected (possibly mechanical in nature). You might consider a cardiac, respiratory, or peripheral vascular problem if the patient stopped to rest. Bending forward at the waist along the way to ease leg discomfort would suggest spinal stenosis.

This simple exercise is valuable for patient care, and encourages use and manipulation of the NeurAxis. Try it along with a fellow student or colleague and compare notes. No wagering, please.

Standing tests

Other more detailed tests to perform while the patient is standing are as follows:

- **Tandem gait: Tandem walking** stresses the balance system and may be tested if the patient is fairly steady walking down the hall on his or her own. Start by holding on to the patient's arm or hand for assurance and balance, and ask the patient to place one foot directly in front of the other (as if he or she were walking on a line). If tethered to a machine or monitor, then have the patient just stand still with one foot in front of the other. Either way, provide plenty of balance support at first, and then let the patient continue on his or her own if he or she does not seem to need any assistance. You can judge and document tandem walking ability based on the amount of support needed to complete the task. Describe your findings like this: Able to perform tandem gait (a) with no help at all, (b) with light one-arm assistance (c) with strong one-arm assistance, or (d) with strong bilateral assistance only.
- **Heel walking and toe walking:** Remember that **heel walking** (ankle dorsiflexed, placing weight on the heel) and **toe walking** (foot plantarflexed placing weight on the ball of the foot) are not tests of balance but of tibialis anterior and gastrocnemius strength, respectively. Therefore, give patients plenty of balance support if necessary to allow these tests to be completed comfortably. Some patients are very reluctant to attempt this maneuver because they are afraid of falling due to perceived lack of balance. Hold on to their arm firmly if this is the case, and give them the balance assistance they need to complete the maneuver.

"Strength was really pretty good throughout, about 4 out of 5."

The resident who examined this patient explained that strength was entirely normal in each of the areas that were tested. However, he further explained that because only a few muscle groups were tested, overall strength was rated as "pretty good." Based on the Medical Research Council (MRC) strength scale he chose to use, 4/5 is actually quite weak. This particular scale is the most commonly used rating scale for motor power. It is nonlinear, and confusion therefore often exists regarding the correct numerical designation for certain degrees of weakness.

The MRC strength scale ratings range from 0 to 5. It was published by the Medical Research Council as a memorandum in the early 1940s to aid in the evaluation of soldiers suffering from war-related

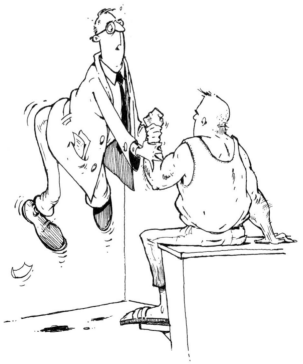

"Your strength seems pretty good, about 4 out of 5 throughout I would say."

injuries. Strength rated at "4 out of 5" actually reflects a substantial decrease of motor power, in the range of 50% or more loss of power. As noted, the scale is nonlinear, which means that 4/5 does not imply 80% of strength is present, and 3/5 does not imply that 60% is present. The scale can be summarized as follows:

0 = no movement

1/5 = flicker of voluntary movement

2/5 = movement through a partial arc of motion with gravity eliminated (not against gravity)

3/5 = movement through an arc of motion against the force of gravity only

4/5 = movement against *some* force (some resistance, although much or most of the power is lost)

5/5 = normal strength

As you can see, if a person is still able to produce **some force** against resistance, then muscle strength is graded as a "**4**," but most of the strength may still have been lost. Patients who are able to ambulate to your clinic without assistance have lower limb strength at least this good. This being the case, one can see that additional grades between 4 and 5 would be very useful, especially in the out-patient setting. This is why many clinicians have modified the scale for their personal use as follows:

4− = able to provide force against minimal resistance

4 = able to exert force against moderate resistance

4+ = able to exert force against fairly strong but not full resistance

5 = normal strength

"What was the pattern of weakness?"

Students are sometimes surprised by this question. Many assume that weakness is always distributed fairly equally to the *entire* limb when there is loss of motor power. As you may already know (or will soon learn), the etiology of muscle weakness is often betrayed by the **pattern** or **distribution** of changes identified during the exam. Certain groups of muscles in each limb are affected preferentially, depending on the **location** (level) of the NeurAxis affected. For instance, the pattern is different for central versus peripheral problems, myopathy versus neuropathy, and nerve versus plexus injury. Careful comparison of proximal versus distal muscles and extensor versus flexor groups will provide important clues to the diagnosis.

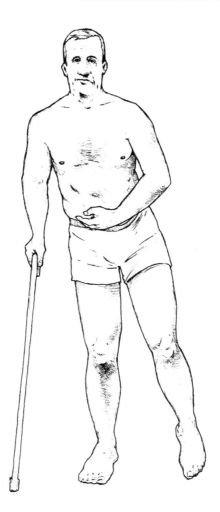

"Pyramidal?"

Pyramidal pattern weakness refers to the pattern of weakness that occurs after injury to (or dysfunction of) the upper motoneuron. The term "pyramidal" refers to those descending motor fibers (axons) that traverse the medullary pyramids (see "Decussation of corticospinal pathway" on graphic, page 33) and is used synonymously with the term "corticospinal." Pyramidal pattern weakness (paresis) occurs when the voluntary motor fibers are affected anywhere along their path from the cerebral cortex through the spinal cord, including the internal capsule and brainstem. Remember, in cases of complete loss of all strength (plegia), a differential pattern cannot be discerned because there is no movement of any of the muscle groups. However, even in cases of complete limb plegia, tone and muscle stretch reflexes will help identify the location of the lesion.

In upper motoneuron or pyramidal pattern weakness, the **upper extremity** muscles that are most severely affected are the deltoid, triceps, finger and wrist extensors, and intrinsic hand muscles (finger abduction and adduction). The other muscles may be weak but should be comparatively stronger. At rest, the upper extremity tends to be maintained in an adducted position next to the body, flexed at the elbow and wrist, with the hand held in a fist. Muscles preferentially affected in the **lower extremity** are the iliopsoas, hamstring, and tibialis anterior. With ambulation, the lower extremity will therefore tend to be extended at the knee with the ankle plantar flexed. With walking, circumduction of the affected lower extremity is necessary to prevent tripping on the toes. The sketch above shows a man with pyramidal predilection weakness due to a right cerebral hemisphere infarct.

Note that this particular pattern of weakness in the upper and lower extremity occurs to a variable degree, depending on the severity or extent of CNS injury. Deliberately comparing strength in the individual muscle groups, and comparing left to right will be necessary to uncover the pattern if it is present.

Rapid alternating movements

When patients report trouble with fine motor control (e.g., button fastening), but motor power is objectively normal, be sure to test **rapid movements**. Subtle slowing of movements on one side may be the only abnormality seen in patients with a cerebellar abnormality, early Parkinson disease, or a small pyramidal tract lesion (e.g., small subcortical infarct). Rapid finger tapping or foot tapping is an excellent test to detect asymmetry between the limbs. Test the speed of index finger tapping against the thumb, and forefoot against the floor. A subtle slowing of rapid movements can be best detected by alternately comparing one side to the other. Be sure to test each limb individually to avoid the synchronization that tends to occur naturally when both sides are used together. Ask the patient to tap the thumb and fingers of the left hand, then separately on the right. With pyramidal tract lesions, the movements tend to be very

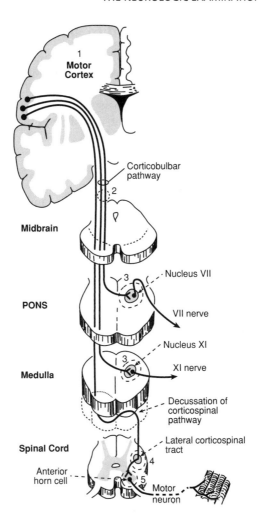

deliberate, slow, and may appear strained. With cerebellar dysfunction, the movements tend to be poorly coordinated with regard to consistency of amplitude, rhythm, and speed. With Parkinson disease, the movements tend to be somewhat slower with progressively decreasing amplitude. A different test of symmetry that does require use of both sides at the same time for comparison is arm roll or finger roll. Have the patient rapidly roll the arms/hands around each other (or alternatively the index fingers) in front of them in each direction and watch closely for asymmetry.

"Reflexes were really hard to get."

After examining a number of patients, you now realize that a particular muscle stretch reflex is either **present** or **absent**. Most students and residents admit that "hard to get" really means that the reflexes were *absent*. However, they will quickly add that they thought that the reflexes *should* have been present, or don't trust their exam skills. When testing muscle stretch reflexes, it is not necessary to use a large amount of force, and you certainly should not strain yourself or injure the patient in the process. Just tap the tendon briskly (see below) and record your findings.

Muscle stretch reflexes may also be labeled **myotatic reflexes** or DTRs. The former two are semantically correct, and the latter is commonly used but considered a misnomer because we actually tap on the superficial tendon. Rapid displacement of this tendon stretches the attached muscle belly, which, in turn, rapidly lengthens the **muscle spindle**. When the reflex arc is fully intact, this causes the muscle to briefly contract. This response is presumed to be an adaptive mechanism that helps us maintain postural tone in the case of sudden shift in body position. It is graded according to the degree and speed of distal limb displacement.

One of the more widely used scales to grade/rate muscle stretch reflexes is the **zero to four plus** scale. Others have been described, but this one is the most commonly used. Whichever you choose to use, it is important to have the proper equipment. A longer reflex hammer and heavier head allow for a greater "swing arm" of force. This type is more reliable in detecting a hypoactive response or in

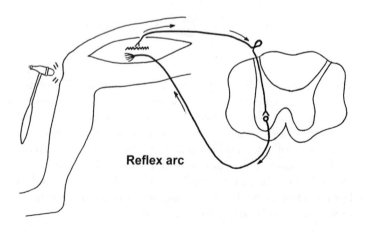

Reflex arc

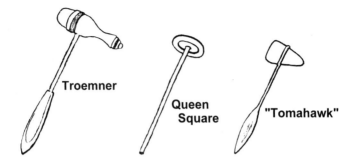

confirming an absent reflex. The smaller "tomahawk"-style rubber hammers do not generally apply enough force to elicit a hypoactive response in larger children or adults, so this apparent lack of response cannot be reliably distinguished from an absent response.

Zero to four plus scale

The zero to four plus scale is graded as follows:

0 = absent (no response even with reinforcement)

+ = present, but hypoactive (may require reinforcement to detect)

++ = "physiological" (normal, if symmetric comparing left to right)

+++ = brisk (may be able to obtain a patellar response even above the knee)

++++ = hyperactive (sometimes with clonus)

"I think reflexes were about 3 out of 4."

Note that the previous respective notations may be shortened to "**1+, 2+, 3+,** or **4+**." These shortened forms refer to the number of pluses for each grade and are described individually in the following paragraphs. The number is correctly reported as a whole number such as **2+**, not a fraction or ratio (i.e., not as "3 out of 4" or "3 over 4"). The scale and notations are also not designed for use of smaller increments between these numbers (i.e., 1–, or one minus, and 2–, or two minus are not appropriate designations).

A good percussion hammer must be used along with **reinforcement** in order to accurately label a response as absent. Reinforcement entails the brief contraction of muscles in limbs other than the one being tested, often combined with distraction. One common method is to ask the patient to look away (i.e., not watch the examiner) while briefly making a fist and/or clenching their jaw. Because the effect of augmentation lasts only a few seconds, the maneuver should be discontinued and then repeated if necessary for the other reflexes tested.

ABSENT RESPONSE

An **absent** muscle stretch reflex is generally considered abnormal, although absent distal responses are commonly seen in diabetics and some elderly patients with no clear pathology/problem. Very mild peripheral nerve injury or degeneration is often blamed for these absent distal responses.

In the majority of patients, an absent response is related to a problem of the root, nerve, or plexus. However, damage or dysfunction at any point along the entire **reflex arc** may lead to an absent response. This monosynaptic arc begins with the muscle stretch receptor (muscle spindle), and includes the afferent nerve, anterior horn cell, efferent nerve, NMJ, and muscle. In patients with a disease

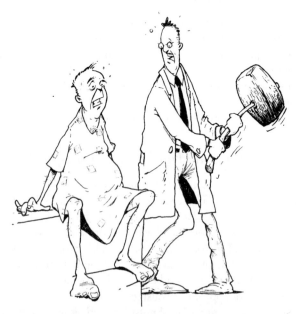

"Your reflexes are really hard to get,
so just clench your jaw and look away."

of the muscle or NMJ, the reflex is diminished if there is significant weakness and typically absent only if the weakness is very severe.

1 + RESPONSE

Use of reinforcement is generally required to detect a **1+** muscle stretch reflex. This "**hypoactive**" response can be considered normal, as long as there is good symmetry (compared to the same contralateral reflex). Asymmetric responses indicate an abnormality, so comparing responses between sides is very important. When responses are asymmetric at a given level, you must depend on other associated signs to help identify which side is abnormal. For instance, the brisk response would be considered abnormal if you found weakness, increased muscle tone, and/or an upgoing plantar response in that limb. These are upper motoneuron findings consistent with a CNS abnormality. Conversely, the less active response would be considered abnormal if associated with weakness, decreased tone, atrophy, and fasciculations. These are lower motoneuron findings suggestive of a problem of the peripheral nervous system.

2 + RESPONSE

A "**physiological**" (**2+**) reflex is considered normal as long as it is symmetric compared to the same response contralaterally. Reinforcement is not necessary to elicit this response.

3 + RESPONSE

A "**brisk**" (**3+**) reflex can also be considered normal if it is symmetric. Reliably discriminating between a 2+ and 3+ is a skill that will be mastered in time with practice. One helpful clue is that the knee jerk (quadriceps reflex) may be obtained by tapping the tendon below *and* above the patella when the reflex is 3+.

4 + RESPONSE

A "**hyperactive**" (**4+**) reflex is considered abnormal and is often associated with clonus. If the same extremity exhibits weakness and increased tone, this indicates a CNS (upper motoneuron) problem. Hyperactive reflexes may also be seen with extreme physical exertion (e.g., during childbirth) and severe psychological stress (e.g., anxiety or panic).

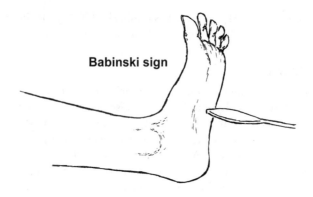

Babinski sign

"Babinski's were positive."

You probably wonder whether positive in this instance means normal or abnormal, good or bad. The truth is that many others reading this note also wonder. You may recall that "**Babinski**" is the surname of a physician who described the abnormal or immature superficial plantar reflex. This consists of an upgoing great toe, often combined with fanning of the other toes and flexion at the ankle, knee, and hip after noxious stimulation of the plantar aspect of the foot. It is an upper motoneuron sign that neurologists may report as "Babinski sign present" or "Babinski sign absent." Others sometimes incorrectly refer to the test of plantar stimulation as the "Babinski test" and the results as "positive" or "negative." The discrepancy illustrates, again, that a simple description of the finding (e.g., upgoing toes with plantar stimulation) would be preferable.

"Romberg was positive walking down the hall."

Romberg is a test of **station**, not of gait. It is not clear what the resident in this case observed, but it is likely that the patient did not ambulate up the hallway with his or her eyes closed. There are several reasons to abandon use of this eponym. It seems to carry a different meaning to those who did not complete a formal rotation in neurology, so one cannot be certain how the test was actually performed. It is also a rather subjective test that is not always clearly normal or abnormal, so a description of the findings provides more useful information. Finally, use of the eponym often leads to distinctions such as "positive" or "negative," which are ambiguous. The correct designation is "Romberg sign present," but even this can be misunderstood by others with a different level of training.

As you know, the Romberg test is a test of **station**, not a test of gait. The test can be correctly performed only if the patient is able to stand still (with good balance) on level ground with his or her eyes open. If the patient appears stable, then the examiner notes any significant change in stability when the eyes are closed. Increased swaying (unsteadiness) or falling suggests a problem with conscious proprioception. See if you find this description helpful: "Station was normal with the eyes open but swaying occurred with the eyes closed, causing the patient to lean and then fall toward the right." Describing your exam findings like this is easy and will usually provide even more information than "positive or negative."

"The sensory exam seemed really difficult."

The **sensory exam** will usually begin as a screen, testing by region initially, and then focusing on a specific area when an abnormality surfaces. Your sampling in each area should include several **primary sensory modalities**, including light touch, pinprick, temperature, position, and vibration. At least one **cortical modality** should also be assessed, such as bilateral simultaneous stimulation, stereognosis, or graphesthesia.

Testing each of the different modalities can be helpful in identifying the location and/or type of neurologic problem present. Specific patterns emerge after damage to certain areas of the nervous system. **Pain and temperature** travel anteriorly in the spinothalamic tract of the cord after crossing. In a hemicord injury, both may be diminished or absent below and contralateral to the level of damage, whereas vibration and position would be affected ipsilaterally. Vibration and position signals are carried to the brain posteriorly in the cord via the dorsal columns. These may be preferentially affected in subacute combined degeneration due to vitamin B-12 deficiency or with a compressive lesion located dorsal to the cord.

In the peripheral nervous system, **pain** signals travel in the smaller unmyelinated nerve fibers, whereas **vibratory** sensation is transmitted by the larger myelinated fibers. One or the other may be predominantly affected, depending on the type/cause of peripheral

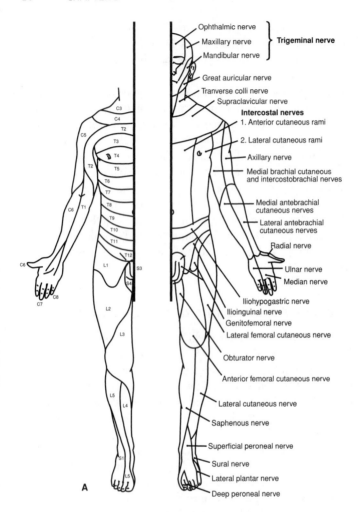

neuropathy. Distal axonal neuropathy tends to decrease ability to sense pain and temperature, whereas segmental demyelination of the peripheral nerves would preferentially decrease ability to feel vibration.

Measuring sensation more quantitatively can be helpful in detecting progression of neuropathy over time. Early sensory loss can be detected and subtle progression measured in neuropathy patients (e.g., diabetics) by using a standard size monofilament line for testing light touch distally in the feet, toes, and fingers. If you do not have a prefabricated kit, small pieces of fishing line in various sizes will do

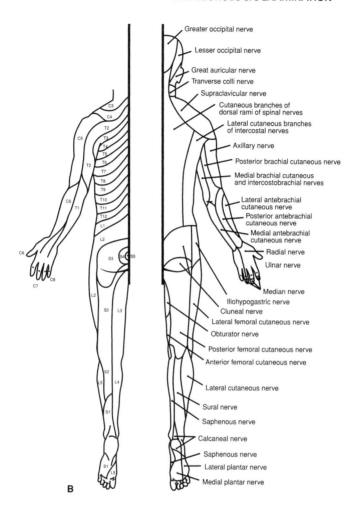

Greater occipital nerve

Lesser occipital nerve

Great auricular nerve

Tranverse colli nerve

Supraclavicular nerve

Cutaneous branches of
dorsal rami of spinal nerves

Lateral cutaneous branches
of intercostal nerves

Axillary nerve

Posterior brachial cutaneous nerve

Medial brachial cutaneous
and intercostobrachial nerves

Lateral antebrachial
cutaneous nerve

Posterior antebrachial
cutaneous nerve

Medial antebrachial
cutaneous nerve

Radial nerve

Ulnar nerve

Median nerve

Iliohypogastric nerve

Cluneal nerve

Lateral femoral cutaneous nerve

Obturator nerve

Posterior femoral cutaneous nerve

Anterior femoral cutaneous nerve

Lateral cutaneous nerve

Sural nerve

Saphenous nerve

Calcaneal nerve

Saphenous nerve

Lateral plantar nerve

Medial plantar nerve

B

just fine. Vibratory sensation also can be measured semiquantitatively by recording how long a person can feel your tuning fork at different locations. Simply document the size/frequency of the tuning fork and record how long the sensation lasts at a given location (e.g., can sense vibration of a 128-hz tuning fork at the first metatarsal-phalangeal joint for 6 seconds).

Remember that the **sensory exam** is more **subjective** than other parts of the neurologic exam. There are several reasons that this is the case. First, patients often experience incomplete sensory loss. Second, there will also be a slight difference in the strength of stimulus that you apply each time. Third, the patient's perception of and response to your exam are subjective and variable. Like motor function, the relative loss of function is usually not an "all or nothing" phenomenon, so comparing sides can be very useful. Be sure to ask if the left feels significantly different than the right, and check to see if sensation is diminished distally compared to more proximal areas. You do not need to test each and every dermatome on your first pass, but a good sampling is required. The speed and accuracy of your sensory exam will continue to improve with experience as you become more skilled and more familiar with the peripheral nerve and nerve root distributions.

"I couldn't do a good neurologic exam."

This student believed that the information obtained during her exam was of no value because the exam itself was limited in scope. The truth is that all reliable data can help us identify the level of the nervous system affected. Her exam may have been limited, but the findings can be combined with information from other sources, ultimately leading us to the correct diagnosis. This is one of the reasons to record results in an easily understood descriptive manner. Remember that with proper training and practice you can *always* perform a good neurologic exam. It is true that the scope of your exam may be somewhat limited due to mechanical factors (e.g., immobilization of a limb) or lack of cooperation (e.g., a comatose patient), but all reliable findings are valuable.

Realize, also, that much of the neurologic exam is subjective and dependent on the skill of the examiner and cooperation of the patient. Like sensation, examination of strength is susceptible to variability, and requires both skill and patience on the part of the examiner. This is one of the reasons that clinical training and practice are so important. If it were not for these challenges, a simple mechanical device could be designed to accurately measure and report motor power possibly with greater accuracy than an experienced clinician. If this same program and data were computerized, it might even be able to render an accurate diagnosis. Because we do not yet have such a device, you will need to be aware of several confounding variables during your manual assessment:

- Many elderly, mildly demented, and/or inattentive patients will require a substantial amount of repetitive verbal **encouragement** before they exert full force.

- Patients with **apraxia** may have a very difficult time carrying out a simple voluntary action when directed to do so. Recognition of this trait and patience are necessary on the examiner's part to complete a reliable motor examination with these patients.
- Patients with musculoskeletal **pain** will often stop far short of providing full force. This is sometimes, but not always, evident when they grimace, groan, or give-way quickly. This common occurrence is referred to as **give-way** weakness and requires some experience to distinguish from true loss of motor power.
- Those suffering from various movement disorders such as Parkinson disease may actually have good motor power but still appear to have difficulty moving the limb through a range of motion against resistance. **Static power** refers to the ability to produce force against a nonmoving (stable) object or to hold a joint in position against applied force. **Kinetic power** refers to a force that is applied through an arc or range of motion (i.e., with the joint moving). In many conditions, both of these are affected equally, but in patients with extrapyramidal disease (e.g., Parkinson

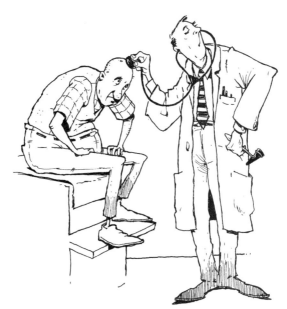

*"I hear a loud grinding noise inside.
We are going to need to order
some very expensive tests."*

disease), static power may remain normal while kinetic power appears significantly diminished.

- Rarely, patients will voluntarily try to appear weak for various reasons. The medical term for someone who feigns an illness is **malingering**. Inconsistencies in the exam can help identify these patients. They may exhibit full strength during one maneuver (e.g., walking on the heels and toes), and then give-way quickly when the same muscles are tested manually (tibialis anterior and gastrocnemius strength, respectively). Repeating tests of different muscle groups, observing the patient carefully in a variety of positions, and using distraction will often help sort out this type of "weakness."

Exam summary

When performing the neurologic examination, be sure to use the right tool for the right job. Check higher-level cognitive function during your detailed mental status exam, purchase and use a good percussion hammer, and keep disposable safety pins on your person (e.g., in a Tic-Tac dispenser) to check sharp sensation. You should also have a nerve, root, and muscle chart handy to be able to quickly check your knowledge of peripheral neurology.

When identifying the area of the nervous system involved, be precise with regard to level affected, and be descriptive when listing the clinical information and side involved. Even if your exam is limited, document the clinical tests that you have had the opportunity to perform, and avoid using scales and terms that are not easily understood. Learn to paint a verbal picture of each patient based on what you see and find.

The NeurAxis Chart

PUTTING IT ALL TOGETHER

*T*he rare conditions in medicine are seen infrequently, and the common ones are seen often. For instance, carpal tunnel syndrome is much more common than thoracic outlet syndrome. This rule of commonality applies to both individual conditions and expected patterns of symptoms. When several different symptoms or problems begin at the same time, we are usually correct in assuming they are related to the same condition. The nervous system is also fairly predictable in its behavior based on the level of injury. Each level of the nervous system accounts for a certain amount of neurologic function, so a problem at each particular level presents with its own characteristic set of symptoms and exam findings (signs). The nervous system is diverse but behaves consistently by level, and it is the predicted patterns that will most often and most easily lead you to the correct diagnosis.

"Pluralitas non est ponenda sine necessitas."

This latin maxim translates to "Plurality should not be posited without necessity." William of Ockham (1285–1349) was a controversial 14th-century philosopher often credited with the supposition, "Things should not be multiplied unnecessarily," although many experts take exception and argue that this is not exactly how he originally stated what is now called the law of parsimony or "Ockham's Razor" (sometimes spelled Occam's Razor). Regardless of origin or intent, the general rule that **the simplest explanation tends to be the best** (or most likely) serves us well in clinical neurology. For instance, if a person is weak on the entire left side of their body (face, arm, and leg), it is most likely related to a single "lesion." You know from basic neuroanatomy that this problem would likely be located in the right cerebral hemisphere. Even Ockham himself (with limited knowledge of neuroanatomy) would agree that this pattern could not realistically be attributed to an abnormality of every nerve or root on the left side of the body (without any on the right being affected). Similarly, it is your basic understanding of neuroanatomy that will allow you to postulate which area of the nervous system is most likely affected given the patient's presenting signs and symptoms. Remember to KEEP IT SIMPLE! Assume from the start that the simplest explanation is the most likely (i.e., The law of parsimony or Ockham's Razor).

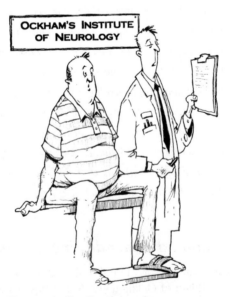

"It sounds like there may be as many as eight different problems that all started at the same time."

If after proper use of this four-step process the patient's diagnosis remains elusive, then you may assume the problem is more complex than first hypothesized (e.g., possibly involving several different levels of the NeurAxis). However, you should still rely on the patient's signs and symptoms to direct you to the next most likely level(s) of the NeurAxis for appropriate testing.

"Where is the lesion?"

Students of neuroanatomy will frequently hear this throughout their studies. The question may sound intimidating, but it doesn't have to be. Start by assuming that there is a simple explanation for the constellation of findings (remember the law of parsimony?). In clinical neurology, arriving at the correct diagnosis usually depends on first simply "bracketing" the problem to two or three potential levels based on the presenting information. These initial possibilities can then be narrowed down further with more focused questioning, a good neurologic examination, and then laboratory testing if indicated. The column of **axis levels** (see chart) consists of ten functionally separate areas. A distinct pattern of symptoms and abnormal signs is expected when damage or dysfunction occurs at any particular level. Keeping the chart in mind during the evaluation will help you conceptualize the nervous system as a set of interrelated levels instead of an overwhelming list of unrelated diseases. Because some overlap exists between the levels, your initial impression may include several potential areas of involvement and will quickly evolve as additional information becomes available. Your focused history and examination will extract the necessary additional information, leading you to an accurate final impression. The **signs and symptoms** listed across the top of the chart are a very good place to start (but, of course, are not exhaustive). They consist mainly of the more discriminating and/or common ones encountered and should provide a sense of direction (guide) when collecting and compiling clinical data. The remainder of this chapter covers salient issues related first to each of the **NeurAxis levels**, and then to the individual **signs and symptoms**.

NeurAxis levels

The NeurAxis levels are listed as follows:

- Cerebral hemisphere
- Brainstem

AXIS LEVELS	Cog-nitive	Seizure	Language (aphasia)	Dys-arthria	Visual Field Loss	Dysconj. Gaze	B/B Incont.	At-rophy	Fascic-ulations	Upgoing toe	Hyper-reflexia	Pain, severe	Sens loss	Weak
Hemisphere	+	+	+	+	+					+	+		+	+
Brainstem				+		+	+			+	+		+	+
Cerebellum				+										
Cord							+			+	+		+	+
AHC								+	+					+
Root								+	+			+	+	+
Plexus								+	+			+	+	+
Nerve						+		+	+			+	+	+
NMJ				+		+								+
Muscle						+		+				+		+

- Cerebellum
- Spinal cord
- Anterior horn cell
- Nerve root
- Plexus
- Peripheral nerve
- NMJ
- Muscle

CEREBRAL HEMISPHERE

Problems in one cerebral hemisphere (left or right) typically cause contralateral weakness and/or sensory change. The face, arm, and leg, or any combination of these, may be affected. The amount of dysfunction seen clinically depends on the size of the lesion and precise location of the area involved. Our understanding of the cortical representation of these areas relies heavily on the work of Dr. Wilder Penfield, a famous Canadian neurosurgeon. In the 1930s, using direct brain stimulation techniques, his group mapped the somatic motor and sensory representation in the cerebral cortex on approximately 400 brain surgery patients under local anesthesia (i.e., while awake). A separate motor and sensory **homunculus** was then drawn along the surface of each cerebral hemisphere, representing the areas of the body that each portion of the cortex serves. The sensory man and motor homunculus (see figures) are products of this work. Understanding **cortical representation** can be very useful in diagnosing disorders of the cerebrum such as stroke, and is critically

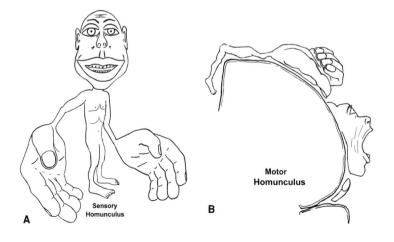

Motor
Homunculus

Sensory
Homunculus

A

B

important when considering neurosurgical procedures for problems such as brain tumor or intractable epilepsy.

The pattern of blood supply (arterial distribution) of the cerebrum versus the brainstem lends to a different clinical presentation of dysfunction in cases of brain hemorrhage and ischemia. The ACA supplies blood to the medial frontal lobe, the area of the cerebral cortex responsible for contralateral lower extremity function. An ACA infarct, therefore, would be expected to cause contralateral lower extremity paresis. However, strokes are more common in the MCA territory, which supplies blood to the lateral frontal lobe, the area also responsible for contralateral upper extremity and face function. A stroke in the MCA territory leads to a distinct pattern of weakness in which the hand is more severely affected than the arm, which is more severely affected than the lower extremity (often with facial weakness below the eye on that side). An enlarging mass in the mesial frontal region can also lead to a distinct pattern of weakness. Because the left and right lower extremity areas are close in proximity, a mass lesion in this region can cause incomplete bilateral lower extremity weakness called **paraparesis** (see motor homunculus graphic above). Being aware of these patterns (sometimes subtle) can help you recognize and diagnose problems earlier.

Language dysfunction is also a very useful localizing sign. The **dominant** cerebral hemisphere is responsible for language and is on the left 95% of the time. Significant injury to or dysfunction of the left cerebral hemisphere often causes **aphasia**. Conversely, injury to the **nondominant** parietal lobe may be associated with **contralateral neglect**. This is a condition marked by inattentiveness to the body on the opposite side. In cases of neglect, you may notice that the patient shaves only on one side or eats off of only one side of the plate. These patients are sometimes not even aware of a severe neurologic deficit such as contralateral paralysis. Loss of a portion of or the entire contralateral **visual field** is referred to as a **homonymous** defect and can occur with damage to the white matter tracts of the temporal, parietal, or occipital lobe (visual radiations) that travel to the occipital cortex. Recognizing these specific patterns of weakness, sensory loss, altered language function, and visual field change will prompt you to test for them, and help you efficiently localize the area of dysfunction.

BRAINSTEM

Clinicians referring to the brainstem generally mean the midbrain, pons, and medulla. However, anatomists will tell you that the brainstem

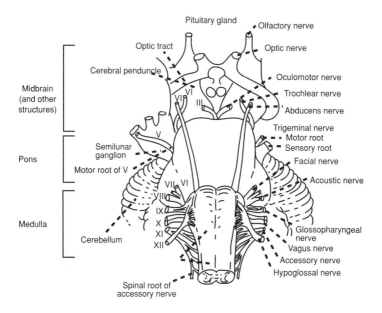

technically includes the diencephalon, which consists of the thalamus, epithalamus, and hypothalamus. For purposes of simplicity, the brainstem here refers to the midbrain, pons, and medulla. A lesion affecting one or more of these three structures tends to cause a very distinct pattern of signs and symptoms. Depending on the level and size of the lesion, a patient may exhibit either bilateral signs or **crossed signs**. For instance, one side of the face and the opposite side of the body may be affected by weakness or sensory change. The cerebellar inflow and outflow tracts traverse the brainstem, so limb and/or gait ataxia is very common with brainstem lesions. **Binocular diplopia** is also common, due to ocular motility deficits leading to dysconjugate gaze. Trouble with speech (but *not* language) and swallowing may also be seen. The nuclei and tracts are tightly packed in the brainstem so even small lesions can lead to a variety of problems such as these. Because small lesions can cause big problems, this region of the NeurAxis is sometimes referred to as "expensive real estate."

BASAL GANGLIA

As you can see from the chart, the basal ganglia are not included as a separate "level." Most of the syndromes related to dysfunction of the basal ganglia are movement disorders that you will see and learn about during your training and experience (e.g., Parkinson disease and essential tremor). Actual visible "lesions" of the basal ganglia leading to a clinical change are not common but are fairly easily recognized. These include, but are not limited to, hemiballismus.

CEREBELLUM

Isolated cerebellar problems generally affect balance and/or limb coordination without sensory loss or weakness. In fact, one of the hallmarks of isolated cerebellar syndromes is the *absence* of sensory change, pain, or loss of strength. Ipsilateral hypotonia may occur with cerebellar hemispheric lesions. Note that brainstem signs *can* be seen with expanding or space-occupying cerebellar lesions due to increased pressure in the posterior fossa and/or direct brainstem compression (sometimes due to edema or expanding hemorrhage).

SPINAL CORD

Abnormalities affecting the entire cross-sectional area of the spinal cord at any level typically lead to bilateral signs and symptoms *below* the level of the lesion. Strength and/or sensory loss (dysfunction) below a definable level (e.g., below the umbilicus) help identify the approximate spinal level of injury. With incomplete cord injury, distinct clinical patterns can emerge depending on the location and size of the lesion. For example, a traumatic unilateral cord injury would cause weakness with loss of position and vibratory sensation below that level on the same side, with contralateral loss of pain and temperature sensation below the lesion (referred to as Brown-Sequard syndrome). Larger lesions of the thoracic cord and upper lumbar spine (i.e., conus medullaris) often lead to incontinence, with bilateral motor and sensory findings below the abnormality.

ANTERIOR HORN CELL

Anterior horn cells (see graphic on the next page) are the nerve cell bodies of peripheral motor nerves. They are functionally part of the peripheral nervous system but are located within the spinal cord (CNS). Damage to the cell body leads to a lower motor neuron pattern of weakness and other findings. You may recall, as an aside, that

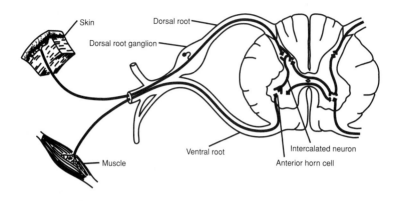

the cranial nerve motor nuclei in the brainstem are functionally analogous to the anterior horn cells of the spinal cord, but only the lower (bulbar) nuclei are affected in disorders such as ALS. The ocular motor nerves (3, 4, and 6) are not affected in motor neuron disease (reason uncertain). The axon from each of the anterior horn cells projects peripherally to innervate a group of 200 to 2,000 striated muscle fibers. Together, the cell body, axon, and muscle fibers innervated are referred to as a **motor unit**. Poliomyelitis and spinal muscular atrophy are diseases that affect just the anterior horn cells and/or lower cranial nerve motor nuclei, leading to a peripheral pattern of weakness (atrophy, fasciculations, diminished muscle stretch reflexes). ALS is more common, and affects both the anterior horn cells and the corticospinal tracts. This disease is unique among neurologic syndromes in that it results in "lower motoneuron" signs (including weakness, atrophy, and fasciculations) combined with "upper motoneuron" signs (hyperreflexia and an extensor plantar response). Again, note that ALS is often associated with bulbar dysfunction, including difficulty with swallowing, but *not* diplopia.

NERVE ROOT

A pair of nerve roots (left and right) exits the spinal canal at each spinal level from the cervical down to the sacral. A problem affecting the nerve root is referred to as **radiculopathy**. The hallmark of acute nerve root damage (or compression) is severe pain. Conditions such as a herniated nucleus pulposus (ruptured disc or "slipped" disc) typically compress only one nerve root at a time. Along with severe radiating pain in the distribution of this particular root, there may be associated weakness and/or sensory change. Other common painful

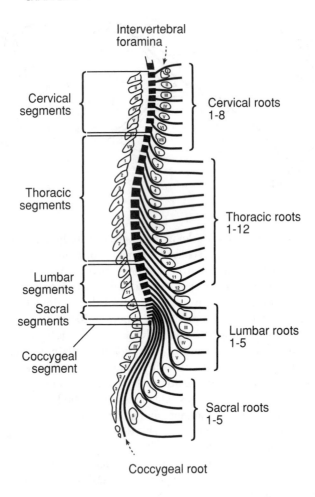

Intervertebral foramina

Cervical segments

Cervical roots 1-8

Thoracic segments

Thoracic roots 1-12

Lumbar segments

Sacral segments

Lumbar roots 1-5

Coccygeal segment

Sacral roots 1-5

Coccygeal root

nerve root problems include shingles (reactivation of herpes zoster from chickenpox) and pseudoclaudication due to lumbar spinal stenosis.

PLEXUS

Each plexus (e.g., cervical, brachial, lumbosacral) is composed of several nerve roots that exchange/combine axons from their respective levels and as an end product form the peripheral nerves. Damage to a plexus, therefore, would be expected to cause sensory loss and weakness in the distribution of more than one root, sometimes combined with pain and/or paresthesias. Trauma, local invasion by neoplasm,

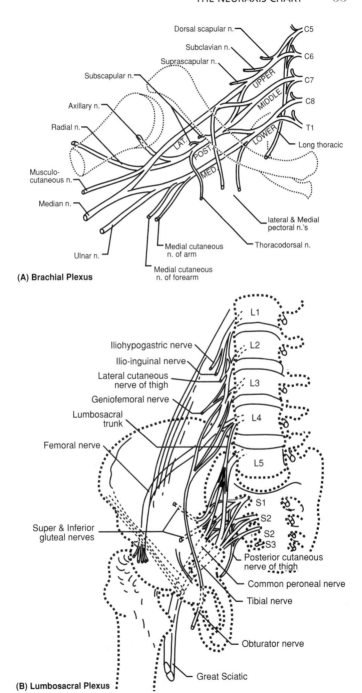

Dorsal scapular n. — C5
Subclavian n. — C6
Suprascapular n.
Subscapular n. — UPPER — C7
Axillary n. — MIDDLE — C8
Radial n. — LOWER — T1
LAT. — Long thoracic
POST.
Musculo-cutaneous n.
MED.
Median n.
lateral & Medial pectoral n.'s
Thoracodorsal n.
Ulnar n. — Medial cutaneous n. of arm
Medial cutaneous n. of forearm

(A) Brachial Plexus

L1
Iliohypogastric nerve — L2
Ilio-inguinal nerve
Lateral cutaneous nerve of thigh — L3
Geniofemoral nerve
Lumbosacral trunk — L4
Femoral nerve — L5
S1
S2
Super & Inferior gluteal nerves — S2
S3
Posterior cutaneous nerve of thigh
Common peroneal nerve
Tibial nerve
Obturator nerve
Great Sciatic

(B) Lumbosacral Plexus

idiopathic plexopathy, and diabetic amyotrophy are among the more common causes of plexus injury. Whether weakness is related to nerve root, plexus, or peripheral nerve damage, it is of the "lower motoneuron" variety. You would therefore expect to see weakness, diminished muscle stretch reflexes, decreased tone, and, in time, possibly atrophy and fasciculations in these patients.

PERIPHERAL NERVE

The peripheral nerves are bundles of nerve fibers with supporting elements, including very small blood vessels. Most are composed of a combination of motor, sensory, and autonomic fibers. Peripheral nerve injury may therefore cause sensory loss and/or weakness in the distribution of the injured nerve, sometimes with pain and/or paresthesias (tingling or burning).

The most common patterns of peripheral neuropathy include (a) peripheral polyneuropathy (e.g., distal polyneuropathy due to diabetes mellitus); (b) mononeuropathy (e.g., carpal tunnel syndrome, Bell's facial nerve palsy); and (c) mononeuropathy multiplex (e.g., combination of multiple mononeuropathies due to a process such as vasculitis).

NMJ

The NMJ is the chemical connection between the motor nerve axon and the muscle. Here, acetylcholine is released by the nerve terminal and attaches to the end plate membrane on the muscle leading to a chain reaction, which results in muscle contraction. Prototypical disorders of the junction include myasthenia gravis and botulism poisoning, both characterized by weakness without pain or sensory change.

MUSCLE

Each skeletal muscle attaches to an origin (proximally) and insertion (distally) via a tendon and is responsible for movement, posture, or locomotion, usually by changes in joint position. Muscle problems lead to weakness, but not sensory change. Some, including polymyositis, may be fairly painful due to the muscle inflammation. The typical pattern of weakness seen with an inflammatory myopathy is proximal muscle weakness. The affected patient complains of difficulty with activities such as climbing stairs or holding things above his or her head, for instance, when placing objects on a shelf.

Important signs and symptoms

The signs and symptoms are listed as follows:

- Mentation
- Seizure
- Language dysfunction
- Dysarthria
- Vision loss
- Dysconjugate gaze
- Bowel or bladder incontinence
- Muscle atrophy
- Fasciculations
- Upgoing toe
- Hyperreflexia
- Severe pain
- Sensory loss
- Weakness

MENTATION

Changes in **mentation** (cognition) are generally a reflection of a fairly widespread problem of both cerebral hemispheres. Common examples include **dementia** due to Alzheimer's disease and metabolic encephalopathy, which is often seen with severe medical illness. **Level of consciousness** can be affected if both cerebral hemispheres are severely injured. The brainstem also mediates consciousness, but thought and emotion are products of the cerebrum. A patient who is awake/alert but exhibiting problems with memory, personality changes, or trouble with mental processing in general is exhibiting dysfunction of one or both of the cerebral hemisphere(s). Remember that changes in higher-level mental functions or cognitive processes can be subtle, so detecting this type of problem often requires you to perform a detailed mental status test, including evaluation of language function.

LANGUAGE

Language refers to the expression or communication of feelings or thoughts by spoken words, writing, or gesturing. **Language function** is a product of the "dominant" cerebral hemisphere. About 90% of people are right handed and thus left hemisphere dominant for handedness and language function. The remaining 10% are either ambidextrous or left handed, and about half of these are still left hemisphere dominant for language. Therefore, roughly 95% of all individuals are left hemisphere dominant for language, so detection of a problem with language function can be a very helpful localizing sign.

Patients commonly come to the hospital because of "confusion," which would suggest a problem of both cerebral hemispheres. Careful evaluation sometimes reveals only aphasia in these patients, and not confusion. When sudden onset language dysfunction occurs, stroke is a consideration that should prompt an urgent evaluation. You will learn that immediate triage in stroke patients can indeed be critical, and aphasia definitely serves as a valuable NeurAxis localizing sign. If language dysfunction is present, then an abnormality of the cerebral hemisphere can be assumed (95% of the time on the left), and the differential can be narrowed quickly. Although closely related clinically, **speech** must be distinguished from **language**.

SPEECH

Speech represents the **articulation** or utterance of sounds/words that communicate ideas. Articulation is the motor action of word or phrase enunciation using the lips and teeth, larynx and pharynx, and palate and tongue. A problem with articulation is referred to as **dysarthria** and is related to imperfect control of muscular movements necessary to make sounds normally. The altered motor function may be related to an abnormality of the cerebral hemisphere, brainstem, cerebellum, or cranial motor nerve nuclei. Dysarthria is a great localizing sign in that, in general, it places the problem "above the neck." For instance, ataxia combined with dysarthria would suggest a cerebellar or brainstem abnormality. One patient recently seen in our clinic presented with quadriparesis and hyperreflexia, but it was her slow, strained speech (dysarthria) that helped place part of the problem above the neck. Appropriate imaging of the brainstem helped rule out an anatomic abnormality in this region, and EMG confirmed the clinical suspicion of ALS with "bulbar" (lower brainstem) findings.

SEIZURE

A **seizure** is a clinical change (motor, sensory, psychical) related to sudden excessive/abnormal electrical discharge of the neurons in the cerebral gray matter (regional or generalized). Because clinical seizure activity is due to electrical dysfunction of one or both cerebral hemispheres, it serves as a valuable localizing sign. You know after a patient experiences a seizure that at least one **cerebral hemisphere** is affected by the process, whether it is hemorrhage, infection, severe hyponatremia, or trauma. When you see a patient with other symptoms such as limb numbness, weakness, or paresthesias, along with new onset seizure, you should initially focus your attention/testing on the contralateral cerebral hemisphere.

VISION LOSS

Visual changes in one field (homonymous) or complete bilateral loss of vision help localize the pathology to one or both of the cerebral hemispheres, respectively. Although problems of the eye (globe) or optic nerve can cause unilateral changes in visual acuity or a visual field, remember that a brainstem or cerebellar abnormality will not. When a patient exhibits a homonymous change in vision (including hemianopsia or quadrantanopsia), the most likely cause is a contralateral cerebral hemisphere abnormality. Sudden complete bilateral loss of vision suggests a bilateral occipital lobe problem (see figure for anatomic detail of the visual pathways).

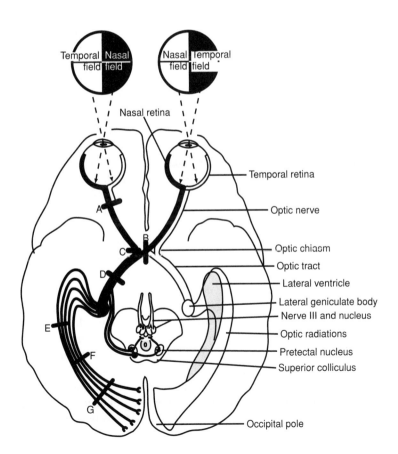

DYSCONJUGATE GAZE

New onset **dysconjugate gaze** leads to **binocular diplopia** that should clear with covering either eye. Diplopia generally does *not* occur with an isolated cerebral hemisphere abnormality. When binocular diplopia (double vision with both eyes open) is reported or when dysconjugate gaze (new) is detected on your exam, a problem in the posterior fossa (i.e., brainstem or cerebellum) must be considered. Other distinct possibilities include (a) dysfunction of one or more of the ocular motor nerves (CN 3, 4, 6) on either side; (b) a NMJ defect (e.g., myasthenia); or (c) extraocular muscle pathology (e.g., thyroid eye disease). Strabismus during childhood typically affects one eye, which turns outward or inward (i.e., exotropia or esotropia). When it occurs early in life, there will likely be loss of vision in one of the eyes (amblyopia) or adaptation so the individual sees objects out of either eye individually (one at a time), and thus there is no diplopia.

INCONTINENCE

Bowel or bladder incontinence implies a lack of voluntary control of the sphincters. This may be neurologic or related to a local or mechanical problem of the urinary bladder or rectum. If nervous system dysfunction is responsible, then abnormal function of the lower spinal cord or cauda equina would be suspect. Although problems of the lumbosacral nerve roots, sacral plexus, or autonomic nerves may cause incontinence, other associated signs or symptoms would likely help identify one of these as the cause. Likewise, when incontinence is associated with an abnormality of the cerebral hemisphere, brainstem, or cervical cord, then significant changes in mentation, bulbar function, and/or limb function is usually seen as well (depending on the exact location). Sensory loss below a definable level on the trunk or abdomen is often a good discriminator in localizing the problem to the corresponding spinal cord level. One recent patient presented with lower extremity weakness combined with an umbilical sensory level and incontinence. Emergent spine MRI revealed a mass compressing the lower cord, which was treated in a timely fashion, saving much of his lower limb function. A different patient soon after presented with rapidly progressive weakness and lower extremity sensory loss without incontinence. This history combined with exam findings, including loss of muscle stretch reflexes throughout, led to a clinical diagnosis of Guillain-Barré syndrome (an acute ascending polyneuropathy), which was confirmed with nerve conduction studies and lumbar puncture.

MUSCLE ATROPHY

Wasting or loss of muscle volume is called **atrophy**. Disuse does lead to partially diminished volume, but severe atrophy is a sign usually indicating lack of innervation. This type of atrophy may be due to a problem of the (a) peripheral nerve, (b) plexus, (c) root, or (d) anterior horn cell. Fairly good muscle bulk can be maintained even in patients with substantial upper motoneuron injury, presumably due to the trophic effects of residual peripheral nerve impulses to the muscle. Patients with muscle pathology such as myositis or muscular dystrophy may also exhibit severe atrophy. In general, severe atrophy helps you identify the neurologic problem as "peripheral." Exceptions are NMJ disorders, which typically do not lead to severe atrophy. If there is significant atrophy without sensory changes or pain, you might consider an anterior horn cell problem. If sensory changes or symptoms are present, then a peripheral nerve, root, or plexus problem would be suspected.

FASCICULATIONS

Fasciculations simply stated are irregular brief abnormal contractions of individual **motor units** (groups of muscle fibers). They can be visualized just underneath the skin in slender individuals (or in areas with less subcutaneous fat). When present, they appear as an irregular rapid and random flickering, sometimes wormlike (vermicular), movement. In contrast, **fibrillations** are not visible to the naked eye but can be heard and seen with the aid of an EMG needle and machine. Fasciculations are *not* powerful enough to move a joint, although occasionally the position of a finger will change slightly with a nearby fasciculation. Detecting fasciculations requires careful inspection of the limbs or tongue. Using indirect light and intermittent local mechanical stimulation (tapping or gentle pressure) can be helpful. Fasciculations imply an abnormality of the anterior horn cell, root, plexus, or peripheral nerve. However, if there is no associated weakness or muscle atrophy, then the etiology is usually benign (benign fasciculations are common). If, however, weakness is present and upper motoneuron signs are detected, then motor neuron disease (ALS, or Lou Gehrig's disease) is a consideration. Occasionally, patients with a fine hand or arm tremor are incorrectly labeled as having "fasciculations." Remember, fasciculations should not move a large joint and are intermittent and random, not rhythmic.

UPGOING TOE

Gently stroking the plantar aspect of the foot along the S-1 dermatome with a sharp object will lead to a superficial plantar response consisting of either an **upgoing** or a **downgoing** great toe. Generally, the other toes move in the same direction as the great toe, either up or down. The pathologic (abnormal) response consists of extension of great toe (possibly with extension and fanning of the other toes) after noxious plantar stimulation. This may be correctly labeled an **extensor plantar response** or **"Babinski sign"** named after the French neurologist Josef-Francois-Felix Babinski (1857–1932) who trained under Charcot. The "triple flexion" response that often accompanies upgoing toes following plantar stimulation involves dorsiflexion of the ankle with flexion of the knee and hip.

The extensor plantar response (upgoing toe) can be interpreted as a sign of corticospinal tract dysfunction except in the very young, where it is considered normal until about 18 months of age. The pathologic response occurs with a problem within the CNS. It implies dysfunction of the pyramidal motor system along the NeurAxis anywhere from the cerebral cortex through the brainstem and down to the lateral corticospinal tracts of the cord. When present, this finding can prove very helpful to the clinician when trying to determine the approximate level of nervous system involvement (remember step 1, or bracketing?). For instance, weakness of a limb combined with an extensor plantar response and hyperactive DTRs places the problem within the CNS. Remember to be descriptive when possible. The **plantar response** is not a "Babinski test," and downgoing toes should not be labeled "negative Babinski" or "normal Babinski." Using descriptive terminology such as "upgoing toes" or "downgoing toes with plantar stimulation" works best in most situations.

HYPERREFLEXIA

Muscle stretch reflexes or DTRs are actually a product of sudden stretching of the muscle spindle located deep within the belly of the muscle, not the tendon. **Muscle stretch reflex** and **myotatic reflex** are more appropriate as descriptive terms because it is the muscle (not the tendon) that is briefly lengthened by briskly tapping the attached superficial tendon with a reflex hammer. **Absent** muscle stretch reflexes imply a problem somewhere along the reflex arc but are common distally with age. The reflex arc consists of the peripheral nerve, anterior horn cell, spinal root, and plexus. **Hyperactive** muscle stretch reflexes are seen with corticospinal tract dysfunction (brain and/or spinal cord level injury). Even mild or subtle reflex asymmetry can help localize the abnormality. Relative hyperreflexia on one side accompanied by weakness and an extensor plantar response suggests an upper motoneuron (corticospinal tract) problem. An absent or relatively hypoactive muscle stretch reflex in one limb combined with weakness and sensory change would implicate a problem of the nerve root, plexus, or peripheral nerve (i.e., a peripheral problem).

SEVERE PAIN

Severe discomfort, especially when isolated to one particular limb or region is an excellent clue that the problem lies outside the CNS. **Mechanical pain** is one common example, and **radiculopathy** is another. A patient with weakness, sensory change, and severe arm pain is suffering from symptoms suggestive of cervical radiculopathy, not stroke. As the rare exception, a more widespread and persistent vague discomfort *can* be the product of a problem within the CNS. However, these patients typically endorse other symptoms and/or exhibit signs suggestive of CNS dysfunction (e.g., upper motoneuron findings).

SENSORY LOSS

Sensory changes can be seen with problems over a wide range of the NeurAxis. Their *presence* helps in at least two ways, by implicating nervous system involvement and by eliminating from your differential those levels that do not modulate sensation (including the cerebellum, anterior horn cells, muscle, and NMJ). The distinct *pattern* of sensory change helps define the exact location of the problem. For instance, a hemisensory pattern of loss involving the face, arm, and leg on one side of the body suggests a disorder of the contralateral cerebral hemisphere or thalamus. Conversely, if one side of the face and the opposite side of the body are affected ("crossed signs"), the brainstem is likely involved. Distal sensory change in the hands and feet (a glove and stocking distribution) is the pattern typically seen in peripheral polyneuropathy. Your clinical impression will be based on this information, and this will help you focus your exam and direct further testing. Remember to examine patients carefully for subtle changes in sensation by comparing distal versus proximal sites (e.g., feet versus legs) and left versus right. Don't be fooled by migrating subjective (patient reported) sensory symptoms such as patchy tingling or burning, which are common complaints in chronic pain patients who may not be suffering from a neurologic problem.

WEAKNESS

Weakness refers to a loss of **muscle strength** (motor power), and not a lack of energy, motivation, or balance. This clinical distinction helps highlight the importance of a complete history and examination. Diminished strength is labeled **paresis**, whereas **paralysis** implies complete loss of voluntary strength/movement. A decrease in motor power can occur with dysfunction at almost any level along the

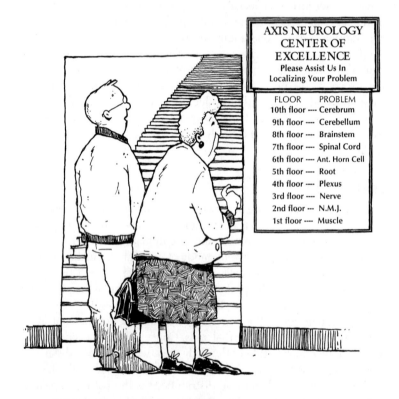

"Uh, Vera...what is bothering you the most, remembering names or climbing stairs?"

NeurAxis, except the cerebellum. It is therefore the **pattern** of weakness and **associated findings** that help you identify the location of the responsible abnormality. Stated another way, the cause of weakness is usually betrayed by the company it keeps. For instance, weakness combined with "pyramidal signs" such as brisk muscle stretch reflexes, increased tone, clonus, and extensor plantar response point to the CNS (cerebrum, brainstem, or spinal cord). Weakness with associated atrophy, fasciculations, diminished muscle stretch reflexes, and decreased tone indicates a peripheral nervous system abnormality (anterior horn cell, root, plexus, nerve). **Subtle weakness** due to CNS involvement is sometimes most evident in decreased rapidity or amplitude of fine alternating movements (e.g., finger or foot tapping, and arm or finger roll). These patients may report subjective trouble with "skilled movements" such as tying a shoe or fastening a button. Be sure to compare rapid alternating movements between the right and left side, in both upper and lower extremities.

What Could the Problem Be?

QUICKLY CONSIDER THE POSSIBILITIES

What is the problem at the affected level?

You have covered a lot of ground and are now adept at being able to quickly identify (bracket) which level of the nervous system is likely affected based on the history and exam (signs and symptoms). Now that you know *WHERE* the problem is you will need to begin to hypothesize *WHAT* it could be. In other words, what is the specific problem/pathology at the level in question.

This list of potential diagnoses should take the patient's profile into consideration (i.e., age, gender, medical history). The possibilities will help further direct your testing and possibly even therapeutic intervention.

A good place to start is a mnemonic such as **"CITTEN DVM."** Each letter stands for a specific category, and working your way through the list each time you are evaluating a problem will help you consider most of the possibilities with the confidence that a reliable system can provide.

There are several variants of this mnemonic that will accomplish the same thing, so pick one and stick with it. CITTEN DVM seems

"What" is the problem?	*Remember the mnemonic:* **CITTEN DVM**
C – congenital and inherited	D – degenerative or drugs
I – inflammatory (infectious, immune)	V – vascular
T – toxic	M – metabolic
T – trauma	
E – endocrine	
N – neoplasia or nutritional	

to be as good as any in giving you a place to start and preventing you from overlooking some of the most important problems that can occur at various levels of the NeurAxis. You can also use this mnemonic when assessing problems of the heart, lungs, gastrointestinal tract, and so on. It will provide a level of organization to your presentation on oral rounds, keeping the conversation moving as you consider the various etiologic possibilities and probabilities.

When evaluating neurologic patients you should be able to hypothesize the most likely diagnosis in each case given the level of the NeurAxis that is affected, combined with the patient's profile (age, risk factors, and clinical presentation). For example, if your

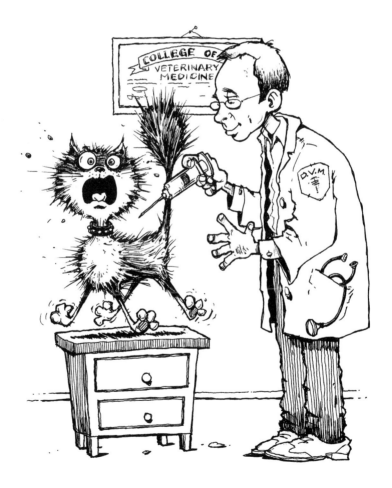

patient is a 60-year-old man with untreated hypertension who presented with a presumed left cerebral hemisphere abnormality (acute right face, arm, and leg weakness), then you might systematically move through CITTEN DVM as follows: The problem is likely *not* congenital because it started suddenly this morning. Infection seems unlikely because there is no history of fever, chills, or sweats. You will quickly work your way down the list until you reach "vascular" and consider stroke (infarct). Based on his age, the rapid onset of symptoms, and your knowledge of neuroanatomy, this *is* the most likely cause of acute left hemisphere dysfunction in his case.

Case Studies

APPLY THE APPROACH TO SOME REAL PATIENTS

You are now ready to try your hand at diagnosing neurologic conditions based on the level of the NeurAxis that
seems most likely affected given the signs and symptoms
present. These cases should allow you to use and further
hone your diagnostic skills while providing some useful
information about a number of common neurologic conditions. The discussion of potential answers follows each
individual case. Be sure to use the NeurAxis chart for
reference!

Case Study 1: "Maybe it's a pinched nerve?"

Mr. Alchemy is a 64-year-old right-handed retired chemist who was
sitting still (reading), when his left hand and arm suddenly lost feeling and strength (ability to move). He picked his left arm up with his
right arm, and it felt "like a noodle." There was no tingling, burning,
or discomfort at all. There was no change in vision, speech, language,
or mentation. The lower extremity did not seem involved, but he didn't
walk much so he is not entirely certain. The sensory loss improved
slowly over 2 days, but he still notices mild weakness and admits to
trouble fastening buttons with his left hand (trouble with fine motor
movements). His grandmother, father, sister, and uncle died in their
40s or 50s from heart disease.

Your examination reveals diminished rapid alternating movements in the left hand and minimal finger abduction weakness. Muscle stretch reflexes are hyperactive in the left upper extremity compared to the right. There is also subtle facial asymmetry, with the left side of the mouth somewhat lower than the right. The left-sided facial weakness appears to be new when compared to his driver's license photo.

What is your initial clinical impression?

a) cervical radiculopathy

b) carpal tunnel syndrome (median neuropathy at the wrist)

c) stroke (cerebral infarct)

d) polymyositis

DISCUSSION

a) **Cervical radiculopathy** certainly can lead to some limb weakness and dermatomal sensory loss. Nerve root compression, however, is usually very painful, and the weakness would be isolated to the affected myotome in that limb. With cervical radiculopathy, the limb pain may also worsen significantly with rotation of the head in the direction of the involved limb (foraminal closure test) and with coughing or sneezing (Valsalva maneuver). The pattern of symptoms in the lower extremity would be similar for lumbar radiculopathy. Here, straight leg raising and/or extension of the lumbar spine may make the symptoms worse. Back or neck pain are *not* necessary features of radiculopathy. In fact, they are often absent in pure radiculopathy.

b) **Carpal tunnel syndrome** is a common peripheral mononeuropathy. You may want to refresh your memory by reviewing a peripheral neurology reference, noting that sensory change with median nerve damage is usually isolated to the lateral three or four digits (including the thumb, index, and middle fingers), and any weakness would be detected only in the thenar eminence (mainly, the abductor pollicis brevis). With median neuropathy due to carpal tunnel syndrome, the symptoms generally are insidious in onset, and typically wax and wane during the day and night, depending on activity and hand position.

d) **Polymyositis** is an inflammatory myopathy that primarily affects the limb muscles. Because it is a muscle disorder, there should be no sensory loss. The weakness is usually primarily proximal in distribution, with distal fine motor movements (rapid alternating movements) relatively spared. Although myopathy can be somewhat painful, any discomfort would be widespread (i.e., not focal or isolated to a single limb).

c) **Correct: Stroke** is the best choice available because you already suspect a CNS problem based on the presence of painless weakness with sensory loss. In addition, rapid movements were slowed and muscle stretch reflexes were hyperactive in the same limb, both suggesting CNS dysfunction. Although you likely considered cervical myelopathy, the patient's facial weakness suggests a problem "above the neck." The presence of aphasia certainly would have helped you isolate the problem to the cerebral hemisphere, but it would not be expected in this case because his problem appears to be located in the nondominant hemisphere. MRI scan of the brain did, in fact, reveal a small right MCA distribution subcortical infarct. Stroke prophylaxis was instituted after the appropriate medical evaluation, and the patient continued to improve some with rehabilitation over the next 3 months.

Case Study 2: "I keep blinking out."

Sarah is a 23-year-old student who is very concerned that she may have to drop out of college this semester. She occasionally has trouble studying for tests because of spells that leave her feeling tired and confused for the rest of the evening. These spells are unpredictable other than being immediately preceded by an odd familiar feeling that she has "been there before" (déjà vu). She then seems to just lose time for a couple of minutes. This has been occurring about two or three times per month since the semester began 4 months ago. Some of these spells have been witnessed by her roommate, who reports that she will stare around the room and pick at her clothes or rub her face, but she does not respond to questions during the spell. Afterward, she is very tired and wants to sleep, and when she awakens, it is often too late to complete her homework or finish studying. She also mentions episodes of "passing out" several times per year since adolescence, labeled "hypoglycemia."

Her complete neurologic examination (including mental status) is normal, as are her vital signs.

Your clinical diagnosis is:

a) hypoglycemia

b) complex partial seizures

c) cerebellar hypoplasia

d) absence seizures

CLUES

Sarah's **loss of consciousness** (or limited responsiveness) implies an alteration of cerebral hemisphere and/or brainstem function. This type of dysfunction may be due to any number of conditions that affect one or both of these regions. Several clues are present in her history that lead you to the diagnosis. To begin, when a spell "comes and goes" in neurology **three things** should always be considered: (i) **vascular "event"** (TIA or syncope), (ii) **seizure**, and (iii) **migraine accompaniment**. Clearly, there are many other things that can lead to symptoms that come and go, but these are by far the most common in neurology. If the diagnosis continues to remain elusive after considering these, a consultation may be necessary (possibly with a neurologist, psychiatrist, or sleep specialist, depending on the story).

Syncope is sudden, usually with minimal to no warning, and affected patients recover almost as soon as they "hit the ground" (assuming they fall from a standing position). It rarely occurs when people are sitting or lying down unless a cardiac rhythm disturbance contributes to the global hypoperfusion of the brain. Clues that suggest syncope include occurrence immediately on standing (e.g., orthostatic hypotension), a history of severe dehydration, or associated certain psychological stressors (e.g., some faint at the sight of blood).

TIAs tend to affect individuals with vascular disease risk factors such as advanced age, hypertension, heart disease, smoking, diabetes, hypercholesterolemia, and family history of similar problems. The average length of a TIA is 30 to 60 minutes, although the symptoms may last hours (by definition, up to 24 hours). These patients report a sudden **full or partial loss** of function (i.e., "negative" symptoms), such as loss of vision, language function, strength, or sensation. "Positive" symptoms such as picking at clothing, limb pain, or seeing bright flashing lights are very uncommon. Typically, those who have a large number of TIAs (especially if these continue for months or years) will eventually experience a stroke with the resultant permanent clinical deficit.

Recurrent **seizures** occur in patients who suffer from epilepsy. There may be altered consciousness along with "positive" symptoms such as limb shaking, tongue biting, and/or automatisms (stereotyped repetitive movements). Sometimes the symptoms such as limb shaking or paresthesias will actually "march" or evolve over a minute or two. This implies the seizure was **partial** in onset with spreading (sometimes called "Jacksonian march"). Likewise, any type of warning such as a strong odor, irrational fear, déjà vu (delusion of recognition), or jamais vu (familiar things seem unfamiliar) suggests that the seizure was focal or partial in onset (even if there is secondary generalization). A postictal state of confusion and/or feeling very tired often occurs after complex partial and convulsive seizures.

Migraine accompaniments are usually visual but may be somatic as well. Although possible, loss of consciousness is not a commonly reported problem with migraine. Flashing lights (often bright and colored), evolution of a zig-zag line followed by scotoma, or tingling of the face or limbs are among the more common symptoms. These are most often "positive" and evolve over 10 to 15 minutes. Headache may or may not be reported immediately after migraines occur, but there is usually a history of headaches. Remember to inquire about pain because individuals with frequent headaches may neglect to mention the associated pain, in part because they are so accustomed to having head discomfort.

DISCUSSION

a) **Hypoglycemia** occurs almost exclusively in diabetics, especially when they use more medication or insulin than necessary or miss meals after their diabetic medication. The warning (if any) would typically include diaphoresis, tachycardia, and feeling light headed. The person would not usually spontaneously recover after just a few seconds to minutes unless given oral or intravenous glucose.

c) Even if you don't know exactly what **cerebellar hypoplasia** is, you recall that an isolated problem in the **cerebellum** will not lead to changes in consciousness unless there is mass effect placing pressure on the brainstem. A smaller than usual cerebellum (hypoplasia) would not cause intermittent spells of altered consciousness. If a cerebellar lesion of any type does expand due to growth, hemorrhage, or edema, then coma might ensue. This type of problem would not "come and go" for minutes at a time (especially over months or years). If the brainstem were involved, one would also expect to see other overt clinical signs of brainstem compression.

d) **Absence seizures** are a specific type of *generalized onset* seizure that begins in childhood or adolescence. They rarely begin as late as early adulthood and are not associated with a warning (aura). These seizures are usually brief (5–10 seconds) and may occur as many as 10 to 20 times in a single day, but without a postictal state of confusion or lethargy. It is important to consider this type of spell in a young person (child or adolescent) because the etiology and treatment is different than with partial onset seizures. The former (outdated) term for these seizures is "petit mal." When episodes of staring begin in the late teen or adult years, they are usually not "absence" or "petit mal" seizures. If seizures are the cause, then they are likely complex partial in type. Remember that absence seizures are quite different from complex partial seizures (see next paragraph), and with very rare exception, do not begin in young adulthood or after.

b) ***Correct:*** **Complex partial seizures** are *partial onset* epileptic seizures that arise from one region of the brain *and* cause altered consciousness or awareness. They usually begin in the temporal or frontal lobe and may be preceded by an aura or warning (which is actually a focal seizure itself). There may be associated automatisms as well, and the spell generally lasts 0.5 to 2 minutes. Afterward, there is often a postictal state of confusion or lethargy that may last minutes to an hour. With seizures, the "partial" refers to the onset being focal, and the "complex" refers to *altered* consciousness (with amnesia for part of the spell being common). Isolated limb shaking due to seizure would correctly be labeled "focal" *unless* altered responsiveness or amnesia was noted. A generalized convulsive seizure could be either primarily generalized in type (generalized at the onset) or secondarily generalized (focal in onset). If an aura is reported prior to a seizure, this serves as a reliable clue that the seizure was, in fact, focal in onset. Most adults with new onset seizures will need brain imaging to rule out a treatable focal brain abnormality (e.g., a tumor).

This patient was diagnosed with **epilepsy**, which is defined as two or more unprovoked seizures (not predictable and not caused by a "fixable" problem). She was subsequently found to have mesial temporal sclerosis by brain MRI, which many believe is evidence of a remote injury or developmental abnormality. Her EEG revealed epileptiform discharges emanating from this region. These tests supported the diagnosis of a complex partial seizure disorder. In patients with epilepsy, however, the EEG and MRI imaging of the brain are not always abnormal. She was treated with the antiepileptic drug carbamazepine (Tegretol) for seizure prophylaxis and was able to continue with her college education.

Case Study 3: "He keeps getting lost on the way home."

Ms. Watson brought her husband to your clinic because he has repeatedly had trouble navigating his way to the local grocery store and has become lost several times on the way home. He doesn't really think there is a problem and, in fact, is rather perturbed that she brought him to see the doctor. He is a 78-year-old retired engineer who has stopped playing poker with his "buddies" because he kept losing track of which cards were in his hand and which game they were playing. His wife reports that he has also had some difficulty remembering phone numbers and even names of familiar people. She now manages the checkbook and pays the bills because of several significant errors he made writing checks over the past year.

Your examination reveals a fairly jocular, pleasant elderly man who has normal cranial nerve, motor, and sensory function. He, of course, knows who he is and recognizes his wife, and is somewhat irritated with her for bringing him to the clinic. He assumes she brought him in "for a checkup." He can correctly state the month and the year, and knows a few details about the current president, but can't seem to come up with his name. When he draws the face of a clock for you, the numbers are spaced unevenly with the 6 and 7 repeated (see clock). When asked to show "10:15," the hands originate at the 12 instead of at the center, and the minute hand incorrectly points toward the 5. He refers to the hands as "arms" when asked how he indicated the time.

You suspect:

a) cervical myelopathy

b) complex partial seizure disorder

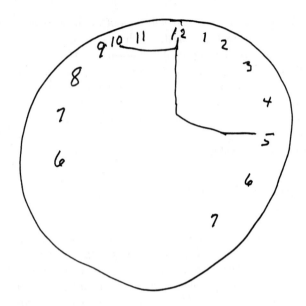

c) left hemisphere stroke

d) dementia, possibly Alzheimer's disease

DISCUSSION

a) **Cervical myelopathy** is a problem that may lead to weakness of all four limbs and upper motoneuron signs on your examination. This would not cause difficulty with cognition, which Mr. Watson clearly demonstrates.

b) **Complex partial seizures** are associated with altered consciousness, but the seizures "come and go" causing distinct but *intermittent* changes in neurologic function (and his problems are consistently present).

c) **Left hemisphere stroke** would lead to weakness and/or sensory change on the right side of the body. Language function may be abnormal as well, with varying degrees of aphasia, depending upon the exact location and size of the injury. Although language function is affected in many patients with dementia, to diagnose dementia there must be a significant change (decline) in memory *plus* at least one other domain of cognitive function (e.g., praxis, language, visuospatial perception, calculation, executive functioning).

d) *Correct:* **Dementia** is the diagnosis in this case, and overall **Alzheimer disease** (AD) is the most common cause of dementia in the elderly. When mildly affected individuals are examined early on in the process, the standard "Mini Mental State" score often falls in the expected "normal" range. This is a standard test of more basic mental function that is scored on a 1 to 30 scale. Loss of ability to perform higher-level cognitive tasks usually occurs first, and this is sometimes more difficult (and time consuming) for the examiner to detect. Historically, the patient's spouse or a close friend will often be the one to notice these "thinking problems" first. The patient may exhibit difficulty with practical (daily) activities such as balancing the checkbook, driving to the grocery store, keeping up with a golf score or poker hand, and the like. More detailed discussion with the patient will help identify other problematic areas such as trouble remembering names of close friends or difficulty with handling novel situations such as a minor traffic accident. Once cognitive difficulty *has* been confirmed, you then know that there is some type of problem affecting the cerebral hemispheres. The actual cause, however, cannot always be confirmed with currently available laboratory tests. Brain imaging rarely reveals evidence of a treatable cause such as subdural hemorrhage, but some potentially treatable causes are not visible on neuroimaging. These include pseudodementia (memory difficulties due to depression) and medication side effects (especially in cases of polypharmacy). In Mr. Watson's case, the MRI brain study showed moderately severe generalized cerebral atrophy, and serum studies also did not reveal a treatable cause. A clinical diagnosis of AD was made, and he continued to progress (worsen) for several years until nursing home placement was necessary. At the current time, the only method of definitively "proving" a diagnosis of AD is by microscopic examination of brain tissue, which is usually obtained at autopsy.

Case Study 4: "We just found him on the sidewalk."

"John Doe" was discovered unconscious on the sidewalk and transported to your hospital by ambulance. He was reportedly found next to an abandoned downtown building. He has no wallet or any form of personal identification on his person.

Your exam reveals an unconscious casually dressed man in his 40s in no obvious discomfort, breathing regularly at a rate of 16 breaths per minute. His blood pressure, pulse, and temperature are normal. A large scalp hematoma is evident on the back of his head, with a small overlying laceration. He does not respond to verbal commands or light tactile stimuli to the limbs.

You can see that he is in a coma and quickly hypothesize that it may be related to:

a) myasthenic crisis

b) a small right cerebral hemisphere stroke

c) head trauma

d) spinal cord compression

CLUES

Coma is a problem caused by damage to or dysfunction of the brainstem or both cerebral hemispheres. The brainstem reticular activating system along with at least one of the two cerebral hemispheres is necessary to maintain consciousness. Note that the brainstem and/or both hemispheres can be indirectly affected by an expanding mass or large lesion of the cerebellum or a single cerebral hemisphere by (a) placing pressure on other areas (e.g., the brainstem or opposite cerebral hemisphere) or (b) increasing intracranial pressure.

DISCUSSION

a) **Myasthenia gravis** is a disorder of the NMJ. A "crisis," as the name implies, refers to acute worsening of the disease and is considered a potential neurologic emergency because the person may lose his or her ability to breathe normally. As you recall, myasthenia causes muscle weakness without pain, sensory changes, or incontinence. Common early symptoms include eyelid ptosis, binocular diplopia (due to dysconjugate gaze), and/or nasal sounding speech. The progressive weakness that occurs when myasthenia worsens can lead to inadequate pulmonary ventilation with resultant hypoxemia. If the hypoventilation became severe enough, the hypoxemia would lead to coma and even death. However, this type of patient would exhibit respiratory distress with rapid shallow respirations with tachycardia (i.e., they wouldn't be breathing comfortably as this patient was).

b) **A small hemispheric infarct** would not directly cause coma. Remember, to maintain consciousness, we need at least one cerebral hemisphere and the brainstem reticular activating system to be intact and working normally. A small isolated lesion in one cerebral hemisphere (or in the cerebellum) would *not* be expected to cause unconsciousness. However, a very *large* hemisphere or cerebellar stroke (infarct or hemorrhage) could cause coma by indirectly affecting the other areas via mass effect or increased intracranial pressure.

d) **Spinal cord injury** at any level would not directly lead to coma. A lesion high enough in the cervical cord could cause pulmonary hypoventilation, but the affected patient would *not* exhibit normal respiratory function.

c) *Correct:* **Head trauma** can definitely lead to coma (often prolonged if severe enough), and this is considered an emergency. Remember to look for evidence of cranial trauma in comatose patients. Other potential causes of coma include hypoglycemia, illicit drug use, and hypoxic-ischemic encephalopathy due to cardiac arrest. In this patient, a glucose level was immediately drawn because hypoglycemia is a common and easily treatable cause of coma. Because trauma was also suspected in his case, a brain CT scan was obtained to rule out a treatable intracranial abnormality such as epidural hemorrhage. The scan was normal, and he slowly recovered over several days. One early hypothesis was that he somehow fell from the abandoned building. Eventually, it became apparent that he was assaulted and lost his wallet and identification in the robbery.

Case Study 5: "My feet burn all the time."

Mr. Smith is a 58-year-old florist with "burning feet." The symptom began about a year ago in his toes and has slowly moved up to his ankles. The feeling is worse at night and better during the day when he is up and around. There is no weakness at all, and he denies any hand or upper extremity involvement. He has noticed some slight sensory loss on the soles of his feet, and they feel "like wood" when he walks without shoes.

Your exam reveals normal cranial nerve function and limb strength. Muscle stretch reflexes are symmetric and present throughout, except for absent ankle jerks (Achilles or gastrocnemius muscle stretch reflex). Sensation is decreased distally in the feet and toes, more to pinprick and temperature than to vibration and light touch.

You decide to order:

a) blood glucose to see if there is evidence of diabetes mellitus as a cause of peripheral polyneuropathy

b) lumbar spine MRI to confirm spinal stenosis

c) serum CK and muscle biopsy to prove inflammatory myopathy

d) brain CT imaging study looking for a left parietal (sensory area) stroke

DISCUSSION

b) **Lumbar spinal stenosis** consists of a narrowed spinal canal, usually due to degenerative changes and/or protruding intervertebral disc(s). Patients with this condition complain of lower extremity discomfort (usually in the calf and/or thigh region), especially with standing and/or ambulating. This condition is often referred to as "pseudoclaudication" because the pain worsens with ambulation. The difference is that the leg pain with true *vascular* claudication improves when the patient stands still to rest. With spinal stenosis, the pain does not improve and may even continue to worsen when standing still. The discomfort is presumed to be a product of multilevel nerve root/cauda equina compression, with the pain being due to either circulatory changes in or direct compression of these roots. Patients become symptomatic with standing and/or walking because the stenotic lumbar spinal canal tends to narrow more in this position due to greater lordosis. Relief can be realized with sitting or with bending over because these positions tend to open the narrowed canal slightly by decreasing the amount of lordotic curve.

c) **Myopathy** can be painful (especially if inflammatory in type), and the discomfort is usually proximal and aching in quality. However, weakness is the hallmark of myopathy, *without* sensory loss or significant changes in muscle stretch reflexes. Both of the latter were seen in this instance.

d) A **parietal lobe infarct** could cause contralateral hemisensory loss (i.e., sensory loss on the opposite side of the body) but would rarely cause pain. An uncommon cause of central pain would be a small thalamic infarct (lacune), which is sometimes associated with contralateral hemisensory change and somatic discomfort. This central pain is sometimes referred to as "funicular pain." It is typically a regional, unilateral, and difficult to define (amorphous) discomfort that is generally *not* position dependent.

a) ***Correct:*** Mr. Smith's symptoms are consistent with a peripheral nerve problem affecting multiple nerves in a symmetric distal pattern. **Peripheral polyneuropathy** symptoms can be primarily sensory, and dysesthesias such as burning and tingling are common. Reflexes are often absent in patients with polyneuropathy, and distal responses are usually affected first. If the neuropathy is sensory in type, then muscle strength should remain normal. Many times the neuropathy is sensorimotor, but the sensory symptoms are reported first. Diabetes mellitus is the most common currently *identifiable* cause of symmetric distal peripheral neuropathy, and this was the diagnosis given to Mr. Smith after testing was completed. Often, in similar cases, no significant metabolic or endocrinologic problem can be identified as causing the neuropathy. These may eventually be labeled "familial" if a positive family history can be elicited, or "idiopathic" if the etiology remains elusive over time despite testing. In addition to alcohol consumption history, a cost-effective laboratory evaluation might include fasting glucose, 75 g 2-hour glucose tolerance test, TSH, and vitamin B-12. Routine screening for other uncommon/rare conditions such as heavy metal poisoning, Lyme disease, sarcoidosis, folate deficiency, and paraneoplastic diseases is usually not helpful or necessary.

Case Study 6: "I just feel unsteady."

Monica is a 26-year-old teacher and mother of two. She began to notice slight difficulty with balance about a year ago, with a tendency to sway to the right. This was tolerable before, but other problems have occurred recently. Her vision now seems blurred on the right, and a month ago, she noticed diminished left arm strength with some numbness.

Your examination reveals subtle weakness in the left upper extremity with decreased finger abduction strength and diminished speed of rapid alternating movements, with intention tremor noted during finger-to-nose testing. Muscle stretch reflexes are hyperactive on the left compared to the right. Plantar response is upgoing on the left as well. Gait is mildly unsteady, with occasional staggering to the right as she ambulated up the hall and with turning around quickly. The right pupil did not react as well to direct light as the left did ("swinging light test").

You suspect:

a) a multifocal process, possibly multiple sclerosis

b) lumbar and cervical radiculopathy on the left

c) myasthenia gravis

d) thoracic myelopathy

DISCUSSION

b) **Radiculopathy** is typically a very painful condition, and simultaneous cervical and lumbar radiculopathy would be an uncommon coincidence, especially in a younger patient. Nerve root, plexus, and peripheral nerve problems (as you know) are associated with *decreased* (hypoactive) or absent muscle stretch reflexes. Radiculopathy would also *not* account for the ataxia or pupillary abnormality.

c) **Myasthenia gravis** is a disorder of the NMJ. Painless weakness occurs, affecting the limbs and respiratory musculature. Fluctuating diplopia, eyelid ptosis, and a nasal speech pattern are also common. Ataxia, pupillary changes, and hyperactive muscle stretch reflexes are not seen.

d) **Thoracic myelopathy** could definitely lead to lower extremity weakness with an upgoing plantar response and hyperactive reflexes, but not upper extremity or cranial nerve-related changes. When considering myelopathy or a cauda equina syndrome, look for bilateral lower extremity findings, and remember to ask about incontinence.

a) *Correct:* **Multiple sclerosis** is a CNS disorder with multiple patchy areas of demyelination distributed throughout the white matter of the brain, brainstem, cerebellum, optic nerve, and/or spinal cord. Monica's exam is abnormal (i.e., there are signs, not just symptoms), with a pattern of abnormalities that cannot be attributed to a single area of the CNS. The afferent pupillary defect on the right suggests prior optic neuritis, and her reported visual symptoms are consistent with this diagnosis as well. Her gait and limb ataxia suggest a problem within the cerebellum or the inflow/outflow tracts (peduncles) between the brainstem and cerebellum. Hyperactive muscle stretch reflexes, an upgoing plantar response, and mild pyramidal weakness on the left are evidence of a corticospinal tract lesion. In this patient's case, an MRI study of the brain was performed, followed by a spinal fluid analysis. Both revealed evidence of multiple sclerosis, and she was treated with disease-modifying therapy to help slow the course of disease progression. Her unsteadiness did not improve, but it did remain stable.

There are several **MS red flags,** and if your patient does not fit this profile then you should reconsider the diagnosis:

(1) MS generally affects a population between the ages of 10 and 50 years at onset.
(2) Ocular signs or symptoms are common (optic neuritis, diplopia).
(3) Bladder problems such as frequency and incontinence are often present.
(4) Sensory symptoms or objective sensory loss are eventually reported in most.
(5) MRI of the brain and/or spinal cord should be abnormal at some point, and spinal fluid reveals suggestive abnormalities in more than 95% of affected patients.

Case Study 7: "I hurt everywhere 24/7."

Terry is a 29-year-old computer analyst who has "seen every doctor in town," and she begins the visit by informing you that "you are her last hope." She has suffered from chronic pain for more than 5 years and has not had any consistent relief from any of the medications or therapies tried so far. Her chronic low back pain started after a "lifting injury" at work. The pain then migrated into her left lower extremity, both upper extremities, and now affects her neck and chest. This "horrible aching discomfort" is punctuated by intermittent shooting pains and affects her almost constantly, with no particular pattern of worsening. To emphasize the disabling nature of her discomfort, she frequently inserts the phrase "24/7" (representing 24 hours/7 days per week). She also complains of intermittent abdominal cramping and "huge knots" that burn and tingle, which periodically rise up on her head, back, and thighs. No medical personnel have ever visualized these, but her husband massages the areas and this seems to help some. All tests have been normal thus far, except for the lumbar spine MRI that revealed a small "bulging disc," which she is convinced is the source of her pain. She has recently depleted her supply of narcotic pain medication, which prompted her visit to your office.

Because she has so many symptoms, you were careful to systematically perform a complete neurologic examination, and her entire exam, including mental status, cranial nerve, motor, and sensory function, was completely normal.

You immediately:

a) order an MRI of her thoracic spine to rule out thoracic spinal cord compression

b) obtain a STAT neurosurgery consult for treatment of radiculopathy

c) sensitively discuss chronic pain management issues with her

d) order a muscle biopsy to rule out myopathy as a cause of her pain

DISCUSSION

a) Because her symptoms are widespread, **thoracic myelopathy** could not account for all of them (especially those above the level of the thoracic cord), and you likely recall that CNS problems rarely cause significant pain. In addition, she does not exhibit objective abnormalities (e.g., weakness, sensory loss, abnormal plantar response, clonus) on examination below the thoracic level that would suggest myelopathy. She admits to urinary frequency and abdominal discomfort but not incontinence.

b) **Radiculopathy** is a consideration when severe pain is reported. However, her discomfort is in a number of separate regions, and the possibility of having six to ten separate nerve roots at several levels affected at the same time combined with a normal exam is very low (remember Ockham's Razor?). Searching for a unifying theory to explain multiple symptoms that are related in time is essential in the diagnostic process.

d) Although an inflammatory **myopathy** *can* cause some pain, this patient's particular pattern of patchy migrating "severe" discomfort would not be typical, and there is no muscle weakness to suggest a muscle disorder. Chronic pain patients often report "weakness," but your focused history will usually reveal that this actually means a lack of energy, mental fatigue ("feeling tired"), or exercise intolerance but not actual loss of motor power.

c) *Correct:* **Chronic somatic pain** conditions often present in this fashion. Multiple tests may prove to be normal or reveal only minor unrelated abnormalities. Quite often, one of these tests *will* show an incidental abnormality (e.g., a bulging lumbar disc), and the patient will convince him- or herself that this is the cause of all of his or her symptoms. This is one of the reasons to avoid ordering tests until you have identified a suspected level of nervous system involvement. When laboratory testing is considered, be sure to have a good reason (indication) based on your history and examination findings.

Case Study 8: "I woke up this morning and my face was pulled to one side."

Mary is a 27-year-old grocery clerk who noticed that her face changed literally overnight. To her, it seems "pulled to the left side," and her right eye is not able to completely close. She denies any pain, change in vision, loss of sensation, altered taste or sense of smell, or trouble with swallowing. Her voice and speech seem normal, and there are no symptoms in either arm or leg. Sounds in her right ear seem "hollow and louder" than on the left.

Your exam reveals severe right-sided facial weakness above and below the level of the eye, with inability to close the eyelids completely on the right. It does appear "pulled to the left" because the right side is weak. There is no loss of sensation, and the muscles of mastication, tongue, and palate are normal.

You believe this is a problem at what level of the NeurAxis?

a) left cerebral hemisphere
b) cerebellum
c) a single cranial nerve (idiopathic facial nerve palsy)
d) the NMJ (myasthenia gravis)

DISCUSSION

(a) A **cerebral hemisphere** problem could potentially lead to facial weakness, although it would be contralateral and affect the *lower* half of the face (below the eye). Each hemisphere provides innervation to both sides of the forehead but contralaterally only to the lower half of the face. Therefore, facial weakness that is caused by a unilateral hemisphere problem is contralateral and primarily below the level of the eye.

(b) An isolated **cerebellar abnormality** may cause dysarthria, but not facial weakness.

(d) A problem at the level of the **NMJ** would, in fact, cause painless weakness without sensory change or altered visual acuity. This weakness, however, would typically be bilateral and fairly symmetric in distribution. Ocular myasthenia can cause eyelid ptosis (usually bilateral) and/or a fluctuating ocular motility disturbance, leading to intermittent binocular diplopia. These signs and symptoms are often very dynamic, worsening with use (i.e., fatigue) and improving with brief rest. Changes in voice, trouble with swallowing, and/or limb weakness indicate "generalized" myasthenia (i.e., not pure ocular myasthenia). If speech is affected, there is often a nasal quality (which may also improve with rest).

(c) *Correct:* **Bell's palsy** is an idiopathic cranial nerve palsy of the facial nerve (seventh cranial nerve). At this point in time, most cases are presumed to be related to inflammation of the nerve (possibly due to a localized viral infection). When the facial nerve is injured, weakness occurs both above and below the eye on the affected side.

Sometimes there is associated pain behind the ear, and occasionally slight tingling is reported on the same side of the face. Hyperacusis and/or impairment in sense of taste may occur if the nerve is damaged before it gives off the *nerve to the stapedius* muscle and *chorda tympani*, respectively. About 75% of patients with idiopathic Bell's palsy recover completely. After damage has occurred, there may be aberrant regeneration of the nerve causing facial synkinesis (twitching of the face while blinking *or* winking of the eye with mouth opening) and/or crocodile tears (tearing on that side when eating). Mary's eye was protected with a patch at night to help avoid corneal irritation (since the eye did not close completely).

Within 2 months, she recovered almost entirely back to normal, with only slight facial synkinesis on that side. One of the potential causes on your differential list for unilateral facial nerve palsy should be **Ramsay Hunt** syndrome. This is caused by a herpetic infection of the geniculate ganglion. These patients report ear pain, and vesicles may be seen on the soft palate and/or in the external auditory canal on the affected side.

Case Study 9: "My arms are weak and I'm losing weight."

Mr. Gardner is a 72-year-old retired postal carrier with slowly progressive hand and arm weakness, with 30 pounds of unexplained weight loss during the past 6 months. There is no pain, and he reports no sensory symptoms such as tingling or numbness. He can ambulate fairly well with no obvious balance trouble but has noticed slight foot drop on the right.

Your examination reveals severe weakness of finger abduction on both sides, with obvious atrophy of the intrinsic hand musculature, including of the first dorsal interosseous on each side. There is weakness of the tibialis anterior on the right and the gastrocnemius on the left. Fasciculations are evident proximally and distally in both upper and lower extremities. Muscle stretch reflexes are hyperactive in the upper and lower extremities, and toes are upgoing on each side with plantar stimulation. Sensory exam is normal.

You believe the problem is related to:

a) left cerebral hemisphere stroke

b) thoracic myelopathy due to a slowly expanding tumor

c) ALS (a disease of the anterior horn cell and lateral corticospinal tract)

d) peripheral polyneuropathy

DISCUSSION

a) A **unilateral cerebral hemisphere** problem such as stroke would be expected to cause only contralateral signs, such as weakness and/or sensory loss. In addition, an isolated problem within the CNS would not be expected to cause fasciculations like those seen here. Finally, stroke would be sudden in onset, not slowly progressive over months.

b) **Thoracic myelopathy** *could* potentially evolve/progress over weeks or months, depending on the cause. However, a thoracic cord problem would lead to signs and symptoms only *below* the level of the lesion (i.e., not in the upper extremities). Other clinical problems often seen with thoracic cord dysfunction include incontinence and/or sensory change in the lower extremities and possibly on the trunk (a "sensory level").

c) **Peripheral polyneuropathy** *would* likely lead to signs and symptoms in all four extremities, typically in a predominantly distal pattern. Depending on the etiology, neuropathy could, in fact, progress over days to years. However, one would expect to find sensory loss and weakness, with *hypoactive* muscle stretch reflexes and a *downgoing* plantar response.

c) ***Correct:* ALS** (also called Lou Gehrig's disease) leads to painless weakness that progresses over months to years. The loss of strength is associated with muscle atrophy and visible fasciculations due to the loss of or damage to the anterior horn cells. The examination should also eventually reveal hyperactive muscle stretch reflexes and an upgoing plantar response due to the lateral corticospinal tract involvement. Features that would suggest an alternative diagnosis (i.e., those *not* typical for ALS) include ocular motility disturbances, sensory loss, change in mentation, and autonomic nervous system dysfunction (e.g., incontinence).

Case Study 10: "He has been very confused since breakfast."

Mr. Green is a 68-year-old local rancher who was transported to the emergency department by his wife because he seems "confused" to her. She explains that he was eating breakfast as usual when he suddenly began "talking gibberish."

On exam, he will not follow simple verbal commands but will mimic basic movements modeled by the examiner. Without this type of prompting, however, he will not even perform simple tasks as instructed (e.g., sticking out his tongue or raising his arm). When he tries to speak, the words are enunciated fairly well, but they make no sense. Strength on the left appears normal, but the right hand moves very slowly, and he cannot lift the right lower extremity entirely off the bed. There is slight facial droop on the right as well. Sensory exam is limited due to lack of ability to communicate, but he withdraws each limb quickly with noxious stimulation.

Given the history and exam findings, you suspect:

a) myopathy, so you order an EMG study of the muscles

b) left cerebral hemisphere stroke, so you order a CT imaging study of the brain

c) lumbar radiculopathy, so you order lumbar spine MRI

d) a hereditary cerebellar degenerative disorder, so you order an MRI of the brain

DISCUSSION

a) **Myopathy** is a disorder of the muscles, which as you know are responsible for movement and locomotion, but *not* sensation or cognition. Muscle diseases cause weakness, cramps, and sometimes pain if inflammation is present. In most types of myopathy, the distribution of weakness is typically symmetric when comparing right to left. His sudden onset of symptoms and the unilateral pattern of weakness would be unusual for a myopathic process. Cognitive and/or language problems could also not be caused by a muscle disorder.

c) **Radiculopathy** at any level typically causes pain, with associated sensory loss and/or weakness if nerve root injury occurs. A process simultaneously affecting multiple roots of one upper and lower extremity at the same time would be very unusual. Nerve root or peripheral nerve injury would also not cause language dysfunction or cognitive changes.

d) A **cerebellar** problem *would* be expected to cause limb and/or gait ataxia possibly associated with dysarthria. However, weakness, sensory loss, and aphasia are not features of a cerebellar disorder.

b) *Correct:* A **left cerebral hemisphere stroke** could cause aphasia and contralateral weakness, and/or sensory loss. Language dysfunction (aphasia) may be seen with dominant cerebral hemisphere injury, and Mr. Green's apparent "confusion" was actually trouble with language function. He was quite alert and attentive but had difficulty with both comprehension and verbal expression. When properly diagnosed early, ischemic stroke patients are candidates for thrombolysis with intravenous therapy or even intraarterial therapy, including thrombolysis.

Case Study 11: "My right arm won't move."

Teresa is a 19-year-old local restaurant employee who reports sudden complete loss of right arm function. She arrives with her mother who confirms the history. Three days ago, after a long day at work, Teresa noticed that her right arm simply would not move at all, and all of the feeling was absent from her shoulder down to the hand. She didn't report the problem until now (3 days later) because, in her words, "it's really no big deal." She has not been able to use the arm at work since then, which apparently slows her down quite a bit and irritates her manager.

Your exam reveals no voluntary movement of the right arm or hand, and no apparent sensation either. However, tone and muscle stretch reflexes are normal, and she does flinch and grimace with unexpected noxious stimuli to the right arm and hand. The neurologic exam is entirely normal otherwise, including cranial nerve and language function.

You suspect:

a) a large left cerebral hemisphere stroke

b) Guillain-Barré, a rapidly progressive peripheral neuropathy

c) carpal tunnel syndrome (median neuropathy at the wrist)

d) conversion disorder or malingering (psychiatric diagnoses)

DISCUSSION

a) A large **left cerebral hemisphere stroke** would cause both upper and lower extremity weakness, often with aphasia. A smaller left hemispheric stroke may lead to isolated right upper extremity weakness, but this weakness would be incomplete and "pyramidal" in distribution (with some biceps and grip strength remaining). Sensory loss due to a small subcortical stroke would likewise be incomplete (with diminished but not entirely absent sensation). Finally, if the upper extremity *was* completely plegic from a central process, the muscle stretch reflexes would likely be asymmetric when comparing upper extremities.

b) **Guillain-Barré** can cause weakness, but this is a widespread process usually affecting all of the limbs to some degree. Also, when strength is lost due to a peripheral neuropathy (especially if demyelinating), muscle stretch reflexes should be diminished if not absent.

c) **Carpal tunnel syndrome** (median neuropathy at the wrist) may cause sensory changes in the hand, along with some intrinsic hand muscle weakness (in the distribution of the median nerve), but not more proximally in the arm and forearm.

d) *Correct:* **Conversion disorder or malingering** is a diagnosis that would fit Teresa's presentation. There are several features that suggest the problem is not neurologic in origin. The pattern of complete monoplegia and sensory loss would be unusual in isolation (i.e., no movement or sensation in one limb in the absence of associated signs or symptoms in other areas).

   Even patients with a contralateral hemisphere stroke have some residual upper extremity strength, unless the stroke is large, and in that case the lower extremity and face would also be affected. Likewise, patients with a hemispheric or thalamic stroke may lose *some* sensation, but the loss is usually incomplete (with some sensation remaining), unless the hemispheric stroke is large in size. With severe weakness, one would also expect the muscle stretch reflexes to be asymmetric, regardless of whether the problem was peripheral or central in location. Note that patients with conversion disorder or malingering may present with a relatively unconcerned attitude despite an apparently serious problem. This is referred to as *"la belle indifference,"* which Teresa seemed to exhibit. She did not even report the problem for several days because it was "no big deal." She was admitted to the psychiatry service and began to improve after a few days with proper treatment.

Case Study 12: "I just can't get up the stairs anymore."

Mr. Chapman is a 56-year-old retail store manager who complains of difficulty walking up stairs. He has also noticed trouble holding his arms above his head to retrieve items off the higher shelves at work. The problem began insidiously about a month ago and is slowly worsening. His muscles seem to ache, but he denies any paresthesias or loss of sensation, and there is no double vision or trouble with speech or swallowing.

Upper and lower extremity weakness is evident proximally with strength graded at 4/5, with only minimal weakness distally. The proximal loss of strength is symmetric, there is no atrophy, and fasciculations are not visualized on close inspection. Toes are downgoing with plantar stimulation, and muscle stretch reflexes are present and symmetric but hypoactive (1+) throughout. Sensory and cranial nerve exams are normal.

His weakness is due to:

a) inflammatory myopathy (polymyositis)

b) thoracic myelopathy due to a herniated intervertebral disc

c) large brainstem infarct

d) bilateral brachial plexopathy due to thoracic outlet syndrome

DISCUSSION

b) **Thoracic myelopathy** can occur with a process that affects the thoracic spinal cord either intrinsically (e.g., a tumor) or extrinsically by compression (e.g., a large herniated disc). Associated signs and symptoms occur only at or below the level of injury, not above. Therefore, if the upper extremities are involved, then the problem must be above the thoracic level. In addition, other symptoms such as sensory loss below the level affected and/or incontinence may be seen with myelopathy.

c) A **large brainstem infarct** could certainly cause bilateral limb weakness, but other findings would be present as well. These would include dysconjugate gaze, sensory loss, dysarthria, dysphagia, ataxia, or possibly coma.

d) Bilateral **brachial plexopathy** would lead to upper extremity signs and symptoms, but not lower extremity weakness. One would also expect to see associated atrophy and sensory changes in the upper extremities if the problem was severe enough to cause objective weakness.

a) *Correct:* Mr. Chapman's history is typical for an **inflammatory myopathy** (polymyositis). His slowly progressive somewhat painful weakness is proximal, symmetric, and not associated with any sensory changes, diplopia, or autonomic dysfunction. After confirmatory testing (including EMG and muscle biopsy),

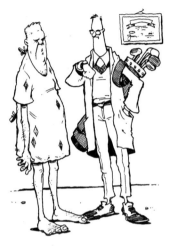

ROCKETSCIENCE
NEUROLOGY ASSOCIATES

"Doc, you look like you are in a bit of a hurry.
Just give me your NeurAxis chart and
I will figure it out on my own."

he was treated with immunomodulatory therapy, which led to marked improvement in his strength.

Case Study 13: "My hands tingle and keep waking me up."

Kellie is a 28-year-old administrative assistant who is having trouble with both of her hands. Over the past year, she has been waking up during the night because of hand tingling. Shaking them helps some at that point, and then she quickly dozes back off to sleep. During the day, if she types a lot or drives for more than half an hour at a time, the same tingling sensation occurs. There is no hand weakness, but turning pages of a book seems difficult now because the sensation in her fingertips is not quite as good as it used to be.

Your exam confirms a mild subjective decrease in ability to appreciate light touch and pin prick in the index and middle fingers of both hands. Two-point discrimination is diminished in the same distribution. There is no weakness, and the remainder of the neuro-logic exam is normal, including cranial nerves, motor exam, and sensation in her lower extremities.

The problem most likely responsible is:

a) thalamic infarct (lacunar stroke)

b) cervical radiculopathy

c) median neuropathy at the wrist (bilateral carpal tunnel syndrome)

d) thoracic myelopathy

DISCUSSION

a) A **thalamic infarct** can lead to *contralateral* hemibody sensory loss if the ventral posterior nuclear complex is affected. This is one of the recognized lacunar syndromes. Kellie's symptoms, however, are bilateral and isolated to the hands and not consistent with a lacunar infarct. Lacune means "small lake," which describes the pathological appearance of these deep small vessel infarcts. Other lacunar syndromes include pure motor hemiparesis, dysarthria-clumsy hand, and ataxic hemiparesis.

b) **Cervical radiculopathy** in the C6, C7, or C8 distribution could potentially cause sensory symptoms or loss in the hand. However, there would likely be more pain, and if both hands are affected, then the problem would have to be bilateral (affecting a cervical root on the left and right). Although possible, this is much less likely than (c), especially in a younger patient. Remember that one of the hallmarks of radiculopathy is **severe pain**, sometimes occurring with weakness and loss of the muscle stretch reflex in that distribution.

d) **Thoracic myelopathy** would not cause symptoms in the upper extremities.

c) *Correct:* **Median neuropathy at the wrist** is a common peripheral mononeuropathy usually due to carpal tunnel syndrome, and Kellie's symptoms are typical. Both hands are often affected to some degree, with tingling mainly in the lateral three digits of the hand and eventual loss of some sensation in the same area. Some patients report an associated aching discomfort (pain) in the hand, wrist, and/or forearm area. Symptoms may worsen at night or while using the hands (e.g., typing, driving, painting). The problem is often treatable with "conservative measures," such as an antiinflammatory medication (to decrease inflammation in the region of the carpal tunnel beneath the carpal ligament where the median nerve travels) or a wrist splint to prevent repetitive or prolonged wrist flexion. Surgery to release the carpal ligament is sometimes necessary to relieve pressure on the median nerve. Kellie did well simply wearing wrist splints at night.

Case Study 14: "I almost ruined my leather seats."

Mr. Jones is a 58-year-old car salesman who suddenly became incontinent of urine while driving his new car this afternoon. He also noticed worsening leg weakness when he tried to get out of the car, a problem that began about 2 days ago. He has had some back pain off and on over the past 3 weeks, but attributes this to lifting some heavy boxes. He was diagnosed with prostate cancer 3 years ago, which was treated with surgery and radiation.

Your examination reveals proximal and distal lower extremity weakness with quadriceps strength rated at 4/5, and more severe weakness in a pyramidal distribution (iliopsoas, hamstrings, and tibialis anterior more severely affected). He can barely ambulate on his own due to the weakness. His muscle stretch reflexes are physiological in the upper extremities and brisk in the lower extremities, with sustained ankle clonus on the right. Toes are bilaterally upgoing with plantar stimulation. Sensory loss to pinprick is noted below the level of the umbilicus (including the lower extremities).

You wonder if this could be an urgent or emergent problem such as:

a) thoracic myelopathy

b) myasthenia gravis

c) cervical radiculopathy

d) conversion disorder

DISCUSSION

b) **Myasthenia gravis** is a disorder of the NMJ, with muscle weakness as the only symptom. Loss of sensation, bowel or bladder incontinence, and upper motoneuron findings would not be related to this problem.

c) **Cervical radiculopathy** would be expected to cause severe unilateral upper extremity pain, possibly along with weakness and sensory loss in the distribution of the affected nerve root. Lower extremity weakness and incontinence would not be expected.

d) **Conversion disorder** is a psychiatric diagnosis. Patients may report loss of strength or sensation, along with a number of other symptoms (e.g., apparent blindness or inability to speak). However, the **objective** upper motoneuron signs (e.g., upgoing toes, brisk muscle stretch reflexes, clonus) suggest an anatomic abnormality, as does the distinct sensory level detected.

a) *Correct:* Mr. Jones is suffering from **thoracic myelopathy** due to extrinsic (extraaxial) cord compression. A pathologic vertebral body compression fracture in his case led to narrowing of the spinal canal and cord compression (due to bone fragments). The weakened bone structure was a product of metastatic prostate cancer to the vertebral bodies. His neurologic problem was detected quickly enough to save substantial neurologic function by surgically relieving pressure on the spinal cord. Diagnosis and treatment of similar patients is considered emergent because rapid diagnosis and treatment is necessary to prevent progression of neurologic disability due to potentially irreversible spinal cord injury. This usually entails emergent neuroimaging (e.g., MRI or CT) and consideration of therapy such as corticosteroids, radiation, and/or surgery.

Case Study 15: "My arm is shaking and I'm not walking the same."

Mrs. White is a 72-year-old retired piano teacher who complains of difficulty with ambulation. She has been walking much slower and with decreased balance, a problem that has slowly progressed over several months. During this time, she has also noticed an intermittent right-hand tremor when sitting still. Her son is with her and adds that family members have noticed that "she just doesn't look the same."

You see a right-hand tremor when she is at rest and distracted during the interview, and at times, she seems to stare without blinking. You would describe her facial appearance as somewhat "masked" with limited animation. There is also a tremor of the right ankle when she sits on the exam table. Tone is increased in the right upper extremity, and motor power is normal, with symmetric muscle stretch reflexes and downgoing toes with plantar stimulation. Cognition, vision, and sensation are normal.

You diagnose:

a) multiple sclerosis (a multifocal CNS disorder)

b) ALS (motor neuron disease)

c) myopathy (inflammatory myopathy)

d) Parkinson disease (a movement disorder)

DISCUSSION

a) **Multiple sclerosis** (MS) is a neurologic disorder that typically has its onset between ages 10 and 50 years, with multiple demyelinating plaques scattered throughout the CNS (brain and spinal cord). Depending on the exact location of the lesions, patients eventually report visual change, weakness, sensory loss, and bladder symptoms. Examination may reveal eye findings such as nystagmus, an afferent pupillary defect, and optic nerve pallor due to prior optic neuritis. Upper motoneuron signs (e.g., hyperreflexia, clonus, an upgoing plantar response) and sensory changes are common. Symptom onset well past age 50, tremor, and masked facies would all be unusual for MS.

b) **ALS** is a disease with pathological changes in the anterior horn cells and the lateral corticospinal tracts of the spinal cord. The associated weakness, therefore, is accompanied by both lower motoneuron and upper motoneuron signs on clinical examination. Widespread weakness with atrophy, fasciculations, hyperreflexia, and an upgoing plantar response are seen as the disease progresses.

c) **Myopathy** (a muscle disorder) would cause weakness, but not tremor or masked facies. The weakness associated with myopathy is typically proximal and symmetric, with the left and right sides being comparably affected.

d) *Correct:* **Parkinson disease** is a movement disorder with a variety of clinical features, including bradykinesia, resting tremor, rigidity, and postural instability. Other common findings include short shuffling steps, decreased arm swing with ambulation, masked facies (limited animation), drooling, hypophonic voice, and micrographia. Individuals with idiopathic Parkinson disease often exhibit unilateral symptoms at onset and improve with levodopa as symptomatic therapy. This medication can be taken in pill form several times per day (usually as Sinemet, the brand name for a combination tablet of carbidopa and levodopa).

Case Study 16: "I get horrible sinus headaches like my mom."

Marcia is a 23-year-old day care supervisor with recurrent severe headaches. She has suffered from them since adolescence, and over the past 2 years, the frequency has increased to about three per month. At the onset, she may notice some flashing lights for a few minutes followed by a severe sometimes throbbing head pain, either on the left or right (sometimes bilateral). The discomfort lasts for about 12 to 24 hours on average, and is associated with "feeling queasy" and light sensitivity. She usually wants to lie down in a quiet dark room, and if she can fall asleep, this helps some. She tried several "allergy medications" with no improvement in the frequency.

Your examination is entirely normal, including mental status, cranial nerves, motor, and sensory exams. Funduscopic exam reveals sharp disc margins (no papilledema), and her blood pressure is 118/72.

After obtaining a normal CT brain imaging study, you diagnose:

a) subarachnoid hemorrhage

b) migraine headaches

c) cervical radiculopathy

d) myasthenia gravis

DISCUSSION

a) **Subarachnoid hemorrhage** (SAH) is bleeding into the subarachnoid space, usually due to aneurysmal rupture. This condition leads to a severe headache, often with loss of consciousness. CT brain imaging study typically reveals evidence of blood in the subarachnoid space. The mortality rate with SAH is as high as

50%, with significant disability in many of those who survive. Having several of these per month, returning to normal in a day or two each time, would not be possible.

c) **Cervical radiculopathy** would cause pain in the upper extremity and possibly limb weakness or sensory change, not a throbbing pain in the head.

d) **Myasthenia gravis** is a disorder of the NMJ leading to weakness, binocular diplopia, and/or eyelid ptosis, but not pain or sensory change or positive visual symptoms.

b) *Correct:* **Migraine headaches** are very common in the general population, especially in younger women. The pain may be unilateral or bilateral, and typically lasts at least a few hours and up to several days. Sometimes the discomfort is dull and bifrontal in location, and feels like "sinus pressure" to the patient. Migraine headaches may have associated nausea and vomiting, light and sound sensitivity, irritability, and may be preceded by an aura (often visual). There is no identifiable anatomic abnormality that causes migraines to occur, and the neurologic examination should be normal or at least unchanged from the patient's baseline. The proper evaluation of new onset headache may include lumbar puncture and/or brain imaging, depending on the clinical presentation. Marcia was treated with a daily **prophylactic** medication, and the headaches became significantly less frequent and less severe over time. A number of **abortive** medications are also available to treat migraine acutely (after the pain has started).

Case Study 17: "I have double vision and trouble swallowing."

Mr. Chalmers is a 68-year-old farmer with episodic double vision. Toward the end of a long day of work, his eyelids droop, and he experiences either horizontal or vertical binocular diplopia, which improves transiently with eye closure and rest. He has lost about 20 pounds over 3 months because of difficulty with swallowing, and his wife says that that his voice sounds different. There is no pain, sensory loss, or incontinence.

Your examination confirms bilateral eyelid ptosis, especially with prolonged upgaze, and a nasal sounding voice that progressively worsens with reading. The examination was otherwise normal, including mental status, strength, muscle stretch reflexes, gait, and sensation.

You strongly suspect:

a) cervical myelopathy

b) brainstem infarct

c) ALS

d) myasthenia gravis

DISCUSSION

a) **Cervical myelopathy** would lead to signs and symptoms below the level of cord involvement, not above.

b) A **brainstem infarct** could cause binocular diplopia by affecting any of the ocular motor nerve nuclei or the medial longitudinal fasciculus, but the resultant diplopia would not be expected to fluctuate this much (i.e., improve with rest).

c) **ALS** does cause weakness and trouble swallowing, but as a rule it does *not* affect ocular motility or eyelid function. Speech in ALS may become strained and slow, but voice is not nasal in quality.

d) *Correct:* **Myasthenia gravis** is a disorder of the NMJ that may be divided into ocular and generalized types based on the distribution of weakness. Ocular myasthenia causes fluctuating eyelid ptosis and binocular diplopia due to abnormal ocular motility. In generalized myasthenia, the ocular findings are accompanied by difficulty with swallowing and/or decreased limb strength. Symptoms in myasthenia tend to improve with rest, and there is no pain, sensory loss, or autonomic dysfunction.

Case Study 18: "I have this terrible pain with a rash on my side."

Ms. Carter is a 62-year-old retired attorney who complains of a steady severe pain along the lower border of her rib cage on the right. It started about 1 week ago, slowly worsening over a few days, after which point a rash began in the same area. She denies any weakness, incontinence, or lower extremity symptoms.

There is a healing vesicular rash that appears to be scabbing along the lower right rib cage. Sensation in this region is slightly diminished to pin prick and light touch. Neurologic exam is otherwise normal.

You suspect:

a) cervical radiculopathy due to a herniated disc

b) thoracic radiculopathy due to herpes zoster (shingles)

c) lumbar radiculopathy due to a bone spur

d) lumbosacral plexopathy

DISCUSSION

a) **Cervical radiculopathy** would be expected to cause severe pain, but not in this distribution.

c) **Lumbar radiculopathy**, likewise, would cause pain but in the lower extremity.

d) **Lumbosacral plexopathy** would be expected to cause weakness, sensory loss, and possibly pain in the distribution of multiple lumbosacral nerve roots, not in the lower chest region.

b) *Correct:* **Thoracic radiculopathy** would lead to pain in the chest or abdominal area, and the rash in her case serves as a clue that the etiology may be infectious. Shingles in adults is due to reactivation of the herpes zoster virus that long before caused chickenpox. This is a very common condition, affecting approximately 10% to 20% of all persons over a lifetime. The associated pain may continue for months to years after the rash heals. The persistent pain is called **postherpetic neuralgia** and is more common in the elderly, affecting up to 50% of those older than 60 years of age who develop shingles. Depending on the level of the affected nerve root, **weakness** of the upper or lower extremity (called "segmental motor weakness") may accompany the sensory changes.

Case Study 19: "Doc, my leg is killing me, just cut it off if you have to!"

Mr. Payne is a 54-year-old car salesman complaining of "horrible leg pain." His pain is so severe that he would rather lose the limb than have to endure the discomfort much longer. It began 2 weeks ago as a deep, sharp, searing pain, and now there is intermittent worsening that feels like a "shooting" discomfort into the left leg and thigh. The pain worsens with bending over, coughing, and sneezing. There is no back discomfort or bowel/bladder incontinence. He can recall no injury or fall and denies lifting any heavy objects around that time. He appears quite uncomfortable in your office, grimacing and having difficulty finding a comfortable position in the chair.

Your exam reveals tibialis anterior and foot inversion weakness on the left at 4/5, with sensory loss on the dorsum of the left foot into the great toe. Raising his left lower extremity to 40 degrees with the knee extended causes severe pain in the lower left leg and foot. Muscle stretch reflexes in the lower extremities are 2+ and symmetric, with a downgoing plantar response on both sides.

You strongly suspect:

a) peripheral polyneuropathy

b) thoracic cord neoplasm

c) lumbar radiculopathy

d) ALS (Lou Gehrig's disease)

DISCUSSION

a) **Peripheral polyneuropathy** would be expected to cause symmetric, predominantly distal symptoms such as tingling and burning in both lower extremities and possibly the upper extremities. Severe unilateral limb pain would not be typical.

b) A **thoracic cord** lesion would cause weakness with upper motoneuron signs, and possibly incontinence, but not severe pain in one limb.

d) **ALS** would lead to progressive weakness (eventually of all limbs), atrophy, and fasciculations (lower motoneuron signs), but not severe pain or sensory loss. Upper motoneuron signs, including hyperactive muscle stretch reflexes and an upgoing plantar response, would eventually be seen.

c) *Correct:* Severe lower extremity pain is the hallmark of **lumbar radiculopathy**, often with weakness and/or sensory loss in the distribution of the affected nerve root. L-5 radiculopathy usually does not lead to changes in the patellar or Achilles reflex because these are primarily L-4 and S-1 innervated muscle stretch reflexes, respectively. The straight leg raising test causes traction on the nerve root, and this leads to pain. Coughing or sneezing (Valsalva maneuver) may also cause sudden worsening of pain due to increased pressure on the already inflamed root.

Case Study 20: "I've been having lots of headaches lately"

Mr. Gray is a 43-year-old businessman with new onset headaches. He reports experiencing daily headaches now for 3 weeks, slowly worsening in intensity. The pain is holocephalic and is exacerbated when he bends over and coughs. He sometimes wakes at night because of the headache. There is no recent change in his general health or medications, and he reports no recent falls or head trauma. He has no history of headaches prior to this.

Your examination reveals subtle weakness on the left, including both the upper and lower extremity with hyperactive muscle stretch reflexes compared to the right. Toes are upgoing on the left with plantar stimulation. Papilledema is evident on your funduscopic exam. Blood pressure is 125/80 mm Hg.

Your presumptive diagnosis is:

a) tension-type headaches (a benign syndrome of recurrent headaches)

b) peripheral neuropathy

c) cervical radiculopathy

d) intracranial mass lesion (tumor)

DISCUSSION

a) A benign headache syndrome such as **tension-type headaches** would not be expected to cause objective abnormalities in motor function, and new onset daily headaches at this age are uncommon.

b) **Peripheral neuropathy** does not cause headache. Other symptoms such as loss of sensation, loss of strength, and uncomfortable paresthesias may occur with neuropathy. Some peripheral nerve conditions such as trigeminal neuralgia do cause pain without any loss of nerve function (weakness or sensory change). The pain with trigeminal neuralgia is usually severe, intermittent, and

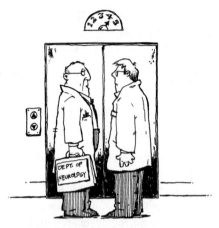

*"They are replacing me with a computerized
nuclear gizmo that will scan the patient,
determine the diagnosis, and then e-mail
a script directly to the pharmacy."*

may be triggered by chewing, talking, or lightly stroking the face. It is usually limited to the maxillary or mandibular distribution of the trigeminal nerve. Similarly, occipital neuralgia causes an intermittent neuralgic-type pain localized to occipital region on the affected side.

c) **Cervical radiculopathy** may cause pain in the hand, arm, and/or shoulder region (sometimes with neck discomfort) but should not lead to headaches.

d) *Correct:* An **intracranial mass lesion** should be suspected for a number of reasons. First, there is no remote history of headaches whatsoever in this 43-year-old person (even tension, migraine, or so-called "sinus headaches"). Second, his headaches are postural and awaken him at night. Finally, the examination is abnormal, including papilledema and weakness with upper motoneuron signs. Mr. Gray was, in fact, diagnosed with a left frontal mass, which was confirmed to be a glial cell tumor after neurosurgical resection.

Suggested Readings

Adams RD, Victor M. *Principles of Neurology*. 8th ed. New York, NY: McGraw-Hill Professional; 2005.

O'Brien MD. *Aids to the Examination of the Peripheral Nervous System*. Philadelphia, Pa: Bailliere Tindall on behalf of the guarantors of Brain; 1986.

Boden SC, Davis DO, Dina TS, et al. Abnormal magnetic-resonance scans of the lumbar spine in asymptomatic subjects: a prospective investigation. *J Bone Joint Surg [Am]* 1990;72:403–408.

Bradley WG, Daroff RB, Fenichel G, Jankovic J. *Neurology in Clinical Practice*. 4th ed . Butterworth-Heinemann; 2003.

Brazis PW, Masdeu JC, Biller J. *Localization in Clinical Neurology*. 5th ed. Philadelphia, Pa: Lippincott Williams & Wilkins; 2006.

Folstein M, Folstein S, McHugh P. Mini-Mental State. A practical method for grading the cognitive state of patients for the clinician. *J Psych Res* 1975;12:189–198.

Haerer AF, DeJong RN. *DeJong's: The Neurologic Examination*. 6th ed. Philadelphia, Pa: Lippincott Williams & Wilkins; 2005.

Jensen MC, Brant-Zawadzki MN, Obuchowski N, et al. Magnetic resonance imaging of the lumbar spine in people without back pain. *N Engl J Med* 1994;331:69–73.

Katzman GL, Dagher AP, Patronas NJ. Incidental findings on brain magnetic resonance imaging from 1000 asymptomatic volunteers. *JAMA* 1999;282;36–39.

Kokmen E, Naessens JM, Offord KP. A short test of mental status: description and preliminary results. *Mayo Clin Proc* 1987; 62:281–288.

Lanska DJ. The history of reflex hammers. *Neurology* 1989;39(11): 1542–1549.

Lanska DJ, Goetz CG. Romberg's sign: development, adoption, and adaptation in the 19th century. *Neurology* 2000;55:1201–1206.

Manter JT, Gatz AJ, Gilman S, Newman SW. *Manter & Gatz's Essentials of Clinical Neuroanatomy and Neurophysiology*. 10th ed. Philadelphia, Pa: FA Davis; 2002.

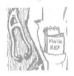

Your Neurologic Exam at a Glance

CRANIAL NERVES (CN)

CN Number	CN Name	Clinical Test
1	Olfactory	Coffee in film canister
2	Optic	Visual acuity, fields, fundi, pupil afferent
3	Occulomotor	Ocular motility, lids, pupil efferent
4	Trochlear	Ocular motility
6	Abducens	Ocular motility
5	Trigeminal	Facial sensation, corneal reflex, jaw strength
7	Facial	Facial, eye brow, orbicularis movement, taste
8	Vestibulocochlear	Auditory acuity, doll's eyes, or caloric testing in coma patients
9 & 10	Glossopharyngeal and vagus	Palate movement, phonation, gag, posterior tongue taste
11	Spinal accessory	Head rotation, neck flexion, shrug
12	Hypoglossal	Tongue movements

MOTOR EXAM

Components of Exam	Major Muscle Groups to be Tested
Strength (0, 1/5, 2/5, 3/5, 4–/5, 4/5, 4+/5, 5/5)	Neck flexion and extension
Muscle stretch reflexes (0, 1+, 2+, 3+, 4+)	Shoulder shrug and sternocleidomastoid
Gait and station (walk in hallway, heel walk, toe walk, tandem)	Biceps and triceps
Coordination (look for errors in rate, range, force, direction): Observe and test finger–nose, heel–shin, knee pat (rapid pronation–supination)	Hand grip and wrist extension, forearm supination and pronation
Rapid movements (finger tap, toe tap, arm roll)	
Muscle bulk and tone, fasciculations present?	Finger abduction and adduction
	Iliopsoas and gluteus maximus
Tremor, dystonia, clonus present?	Quadriceps and hamstring
Plantar response	Tibialis anterior and gastrocnemius

SENSORY EXAM

Modalities to be Tested (See Dermatome Chart)
Sharp (pin)
Light touch (paper towel, cotton)
Temperature (cool tuning fork)
Vibration (tuning fork)
Position (large toe, finger)
Cortical (simultaneous, graphesthesia)

MENTAL STATUS EXAM

Components of Exam	Examples/Suggestions
Orientation	Oriented to place, time (day/month/year), person (knows relationship of others such as nurse, brother, wife), "oriented ×4" means also oriented for reason for being at clinic or in hospital
Fund of knowledge and intellect	Discuss current newsworthy events, compare/contrast recent presidents, sports teams, plants, foods, name last five presidents, name five major U.S. or international cities
Language function	Verbal fluency and receptive language function: speak, read, write a sentence or two, understand two- to three-step commands, look for paraphasic errors saying phrase such as "no ifs, ands, or buts" or "methodist episcopal"
Abstract phrases	Proverbs: Stitch in time, spilled milk, bird in the hand; Similarities: apple–banana, car–plane, table–chair
Clock drawing test	Face of clock with numbers, indicate 10:15 (no further directions)
Judgment	Give a novel more complex "what would you do . . ." scenario (e.g., if involved in a minor traffic accident on a dark street)
Short-term memory	Have patient register three unrelated objects and recall in 2–3 minutes
Concentration	Spell WORLD forward then backward, perform serial 7s or 3s
Calculations	Give simple, then more complex mental calculations
Praxis	Have patient show how (pretend) to use a comb, flip a coin, drink from a straw
Affect, attentiveness, sense of humor	Appearance, response time, smile, laughing appropriately (describe level of consciousness also, especially in hospitalized patients)
Thought processes	Listen for loose associations, flight of ideas, racing, tangential, circumstantial, irrelevance
Thought content	Delusions, hallucinations, obsessions, compulsions, phobias, suicidal

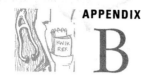

The NeurAxis Chart

AXIS LEVELS	Cog-nitive	Seizure	Language (aphasia)	Dys-arthria	Visual Field Loss	Dysconj. Gaze	B/B Incont.	At-rophy	Fascic-ulations	Upgoing toe	Hyper-reflexia	Pain, severe	Sens loss	Weak
Hemisphere	+	+	+	+	+					+	+		+	+
Brainstem				+		+	+			+	+		+	+
Cerebellum				+										
Cord							+			+	+		+	+
AHC								+	+					+
Root								+	+			+	+	+
Plexus								+	+			+	+	+
Nerve						+		+	+			+	+	+
NMJ				+		+								+
Muscle						+		+				+		+

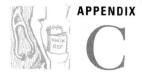

APPENDIX

C

Did You Know?

ALS (also known as Lou Gehrig's disease): In 1995, Cal Ripken, a Baltimore Orioles shortstop known as the "Iron Man," broke Lou Gehrig's amazing record of 2,130 consecutive games played. Gehrig himself was known as the "Iron Horse" for his resiliency prior to developing ALS and retiring from baseball after his emotional "luckiest man" address to Yankee fans in 1939. Ripken went on to play in 2,632 consecutive games, voluntarily sitting out his streak-ending game in 1998 while his team played the late Gehrig's New York Yankees.

HOMUNCULUS: Our understanding of the cortical representation of these areas depends heavily on the work of Dr. Wilder Penfield, a famous Canadian neurosurgeon. In the 1930s, using direct brain stimulation, he actually mapped the somatic motor and sensory representation in the cerebral cortex on approximately 400 brain surgery patients under local anesthesia (i.e., while awake). A **homunculus** was then drawn along the surface of each cerebral hemisphere, representing the areas of the body that each portion of the cortex serves (see figure on page 49). As a matter of interest, around the time of Paracelcius (1493–1541), it was believed by some that a small homunculus (man) could be produced by incubating human semen within a dunghill.

REFLEX HAMMER: The current-day **reflex hammer** has been widely used as such since the late 1800s, when the clinical utility of muscle stretch reflexes was described by Wilhelm H. Erb and Karl Westphal. Prior to that, a similar instrument had been used as a **chest percussion hammer**, an instrument adapted from the tool used by ranchers to percuss animal skulls in search of possible hydatid cysts inside. The concept of percussing as a useful medical test appears to have originated with the observation that thumping wine casks could define the fluid level inside.

111

ROMBERG: The modern **Romberg test** evolved after the description (by several physicians in the early 19th century, including Dr. Moritz Romberg) of postural instability that worsened in the dark. Romberg published his accounts of the sign in the mid-1800s and considered it diagnostic of tabes dorsalis.

Index

Page numbers followed by f indicate figures.